Fight Parkinson's and Huntington's with Vitamins and Antioxidants

Kedar N. Prasad, Ph.D.

Healing Arts Press
Rochester, Vermont • Toronto, Canada

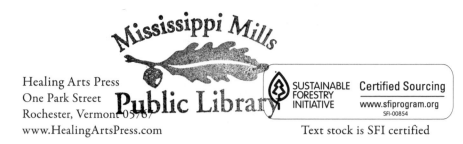

Healing Arts Press
One Park Street
Rochester, Vermont 05767
www.HealingArtsPress.com

SUSTAINABLE FORESTRY INITIATIVE
Certified Sourcing
www.sfiprogram.org
SFI-00854

Text stock is SFI certified

Healing Arts Press is a division of Inner Traditions International

Note to the reader: *This book is intended as an informational guide. The remedies, approaches, and techniques described herein are meant to supplement, and not to be a substitute for, professional medical care or treatment. They should not be used to treat a serious ailment without prior consultation with a qualified health care professional.*

Library of Congress Cataloging-in-Publication Data

Names: Prasad, Kedar N., author.
Title: Fight Parkinson's and Huntington's with vitamins and antioxidants / Kedar N. Prasad.
Description: Rochester, Vermont : Healing Arts Press, [2016] | Includes bibliographical references and index.
Identifiers: LCCN 2015036573| ISBN 9781620554333 (paperback) | ISBN 9781620554340 (e-book)
Subjects: LCSH: Parkinson's disease--Diet therapy. | Huntington's disease—Diet therapy. | Vitamin therapy. | Antioxidants—Therapeutic use. | BISAC: HEALTH & FITNESS / Vitamins. | MEDICAL / Diseases. | HEALTH & FITNESS / Diseases / Nervous System (incl. Brain).
Classification: LCC RC382 .P73 2016 | DDC 616.8/3306—dc23
LC record available at http://lccn.loc.gov/2015036573

Printed and bound in the United States by Lake Book Manufacturing, Inc. The text stock is SFI certified. The Sustainable Forestry Initiative® program promotes sustainable forest management.

10 9 8 7 6 5 4 3 2 1

Text design by Virginia Scott Bowman and layout by Priscilla Baker
This book was typeset in Garamond Premier Pro with Helvetica Neue used as a display typeface

To send correspondence to the author of this book, mail a first-class letter to the author c/o Inner Traditions • Bear & Company, One Park Street, Rochester, VT 05767, and we will forward the communication, or contact the author directly at **knprasad@comcast.net**.

Contents

■ ■ ■

ACKNOWLEDGMENTS

I would like to thank my family for their support and encouragement. I also am very thankful to Anne Dillon and Chanc VanWinkle Orzell for their superb editing of this book.

Why Should You Read This Book?

Although humankind suffers many neurological diseases, this book focuses on the neurodegenerative Parkinson's disease and Huntington's disease. About 1 million people suffer from Parkinson's disease, with about 60,000 new cases diagnosed annually in the USA and 3 million to 4 million people remaining undiagnosed. Huntington's disease, on the other hand, is estimated to have an incidence of about 1,500 per year.

The direct and indirect cost of Parkinson's disease is estimated to be about $25 billion per year, while the annual cost of treating Huntington's disease may vary. The average annual medical cost per individual is about $10,500, but it could be as much as $47,000 if caregivers' costs are included.

Parkinson's disease is considered a slow, progressive chronic neuro-degenerative disease appearing later in life and characterized by the loss of dopamine neurons from the brain, which causes involuntary tremors of the limbs and trunk as well as non-motor deficits and neurological symptoms, including impaired sense of smell, memory loss, and psychiatric symptoms. Parkinson's is the most common form of neurodegenerative disease after Alzheimer's disease.

In contrast, symptoms of Huntington's disease—an incurable and fatal genetic disease caused by a gene mutation—appear in young adult life and become progressively worse. The major symptoms of Huntington's include movement disorders, cognitive dysfunction, and psychiatric problems. The movement disorders are characterized by uncontrolled movement or tics in the fingers, feet, face, or trunk, which become more intense when the individuals are anxious or disturbed. As the disease progresses, other symptoms appear, such as clumsiness, jaw clenching (bruxism), loss of coordination and balance, slurred speech, difficulty swallowing and eating, uncontrolled continual muscular contractions (dystonia), difficulty walking, stumbling, and falling. The cognitive dysfunctions are characterized by progressive loss of memory, including the ability to concentrate, answer questions, and recognize familiar objects.

At present, there is no adequate strategy for the prevention of Parkinson's disease and the mitigation of Huntington's disease symptoms, and their treatment options remain unsatisfactory. In this book I propose a unified hypothesis that increased oxidative stress and chronic inflammation are primarily responsible for the initiation and progression of these diseases. Therefore, mitigating oxidative stress and chronic inflammation appears to be a logical solution to reduce development or progression in both. The proposed strategy, in combination with standard therapy, may improve management outcomes more than just standard therapy alone.

To reduce oxidative stress and chronic inflammation it's essential to increase the body's levels of all antioxidant enzymes and all standard dietary and endogenous antioxidants. This goal cannot be achieved by the use of the one or two antioxidants that have been used in clinical studies. Therefore, I have proposed that a preparation of micronutrients containing *multiple* dietary and endogenous antioxidants, B vitamins with high doses of vitamin B_3 (nicotinamide), vitamin D_3, selenium, and certain polyphenolic compounds (curcumin and resveratrol) should be employed in clinical studies to reduce the risk of development and/or progression of Parkinson's and Huntington's. These micronutrients are capable of increasing the levels of all antioxidant enzymes by activating a nuclear transcriptional factor 2/antioxidant response element (Nrf2/ARE) pathway, as well as by enhancing the levels of standard dietary and endogenous antioxidants.

Even though some laboratory data exist to suggest that even the genetic basis of neurological disease can be prevented or delayed by micronutrient supplements, the increase in the amount of micronutrients that I propose flies in the face of conventional theory, for most neurologists believe that antioxidants and vitamins have no significant role in the prevention or improved management of neurodegenerative diseases. These beliefs are primarily based on a few clinical studies in which supplementation with a single antioxidant, such as coenzyme Q10 in Parkinson's disease, produced only modest beneficial effects in the study group. Another study demonstrated that vitamin E alone was ineffective in reducing the progression of Parkinson's disease.

The fact of the matter is that patients with neurodegenerative diseases may have a high oxidative environment in the brain; thus the administration of a single antioxidant *should not be expected* to produce any significant beneficial effects. This is due to the fact that an individual antioxidant in the presence of a high oxidative environment may be oxidized and then act as a prooxidant rather than as an antioxidant. Also, the levels of the oxidized form of an antioxidant may increase after the prolonged consumption of a single antioxidant; this can subsequently damage brain cells. Coupled with this is the fact that a single antioxidant cannot elevate *all* antioxidant enzymes as well as a multitude of dietary and endogenous antioxidants.

I have published several reviews in peer-reviewed journals challenging the current trends of using a single antioxidant in the prevention and improved management of neurodegenerative diseases in high-risk populations. These articles have failed to have any significant impact on the design of relevant clinical trials, and the inconsistent results of the effects of a single antioxidant continue to be published. The growing controversies regarding the value of multiple micronutrients in the prevention and improved management of neurodegenerative diseases needs to be addressed, and new solutions need to be proposed.

This book describes the reasons for the present controversies and proposes evidence and solutions—that are firmly grounded in scientific rationale—to employ to prevent and improve the management of neurological diseases. Books on neurodegenerative diseases and their causes and symptoms are available; however, none of them have critically analyzed the published data on antioxidants' effects on neurodegenerative diseases. Additionally, none have questioned whether the experimental designs of the studies on which the conclusions were based were scientifically valid, whether the results obtained from the use of a single antioxidant in high-risk populations can be extrapolated to the effect of the same antioxidant in a multiple antioxidant preparation for the same population, or whether the results of studies obtained on high-risk populations can be extrapolated to normal populations. A comprehensive preparation of micronutrients to prevent and improve the management of neurodegenerative diseases has never been proposed. I have done so in this book.

I also discuss oxidative stress, inflammation, properties and function of antioxidants and certain phenolic compounds, structure and function of a normal human brain, and incidence, cost, and causes of each neurodegenerative disease. In addition, I present evidence in support of a hypothesis that increased oxidative stress and chronic inflammation in the brain play an important role in the initiation and progression of Parkinson's and Huntington's disease. Finally, I provide formulations of micronutrients containing multiple dietary and endogenous antioxidants and B vitamins, vitamin D, selenium, and certain polyphenolic compounds (curcumin and resveratrol) specific to each neurodegenerative disease and give recommendations for their prevention and management.

Primary care physicians and practicing neurologists interested in complementary medicine will find this book useful in recommending micronutrient supplements to their patients. I hope that it will also serve as a guide to those afflicted with Parkinson's or Huntington's disease and that those who are taking daily supplements will be comforted by the information provided. Those who are not taking supplements or are uncertain as to their potential benefits may find evidence to help them make a decision as to whether to take micronutrient supplements, in consultation with their doctors. My ultimate goal is to provide hope for a new strategy in mitigating the effects of these serious conditions and to improve the lives of those who suffer from them.

1 A Closer Look at the Human Brain

Despite extensive research by neuroanatomists, neurobiologists, neurochemists, and neurophysiologists, many aspects of the brain's structure and functioning remain tantalizingly unclear. The "Decade of the Brain," an initiative of the U.S. government in the 1990s under President George Bush, has increased our knowledge of brain functioning somewhat. Still, the work goes on to discover its myriad mysteries. Research endeavors include the study of animal and human neuronal and glial cell culture, the brain tissue of animals (primarily rodents and occasionally nonhuman primates), and human brains obtained at autopsy. Current research also includes noninvasive techniques such as electroencephalography (EEG) and functional magnetic resonance imaging (fMRI), as well as invasive techniques such as obtaining fresh brain tissues from animals after euthanasia and human brain samples obtained whenever possible during surgery.

This chapter describes very briefly, and in simple terms, the structure and functions of the human brain that are relevant to chronic neurological diseases. It's important to have a fundamental understanding of how the brain works so that we can better understand the dynamics involved when it becomes impaired.

THE HUMAN BRAIN

Basic Facts

The average weight of the human adult brain is about three pounds (1.5 kilograms). In women the volume of the brain is approximately 1,130 cubic centimeters and in men it is about 1,260 cubic centimeters, although significant individual variations are found. The brain consists of three main regions: the forebrain, midbrain, and hindbrain. Brain regions are divided into the cerebrum, the cerebellum, the limbic system, and the brain stem.

The brain also contains four interconnected cavities that are filled with cerebrospinal fluid, as well as approximately 100 billion neurons.

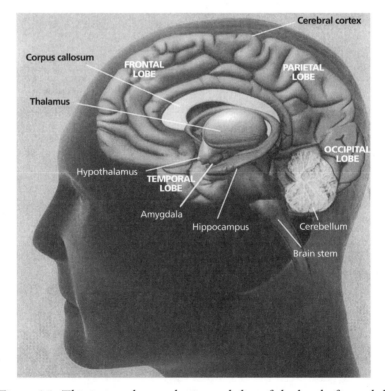

Figure 1.1. This image shows a horizontal slice of the head of an adult man, revealing the different structures of the human brain. Courtesy of the National Library of Medicine's Visible Human Project.

Neurons are a unique type of cell in that they can receive, synthesize, store, and transmit information from one neuron to another. Figure 1.1 presents a view of various structures of the human brain.

The Cerebrum and Its Function

The cerebrum, or cortex, is the largest part of the human brain, having a surface area of about 1.3 square feet ($0.12m^2$), folded in such a way so as to allow it to fit within the skull. This folding causes ridges of the cerebrum; these are called gyri collectively or gyrus in the singular. Crevices in the cortex are called sulcus or sulci (collectively). The cerebrum is divided into the right and left hemispheres, which are connected by a fibrous band of nerves called the corpus callosum. The corpus callosum is responsible for communication between the hemispheres. The right hemisphere controls the left side of the body and oversees temporal and spatial relationships, the analysis of nonverbal information, and the communication of emotion. The left hemisphere controls the right side of the body and produces and understands language.

The cortex of each hemisphere is divided into four lobes: the frontal lobe, the parietal lobe, the occipital lobe, and the temporal lobe. Certain functions of the lobes overlap with one another. The frontal lobe is responsible for cognition and memory, behavior, abstract thought processes, problem solving, analytic and critical reasoning, attention, creative thought, voluntary motor activity, language skills, emotional traits, intellect, reflection, judgment, physical reaction, inhibition, libido (the sexual urge), and initiative.

The parietal lobe oversees basic sensations such as touch, pain, pressure, temperature sensitivity, various joint movements, tactile sensations, spatial relationships, and sensitivity to an exact point of tactile contact as well as the ability to distinguish between two points of tactile stimulation, some language and reading functions, and some visual functions.

The occipital lobe is involved in interpreting visual impulses and reading.

The temporal lobe is involved with auditory (sound) sensations, speech, the sensation of smell, one's sense of identity, fear, music, some vision pathways, and some emotions and memories.

Nerve cells form the gray surface of the cerebrum, which is a little thicker than the nerve fibers that carry signals between nerve cells and other parts of the body.

The Cerebellum

The cerebellum is much smaller than the cerebrum, but, like the cerebrum, it has a highly folded surface. This portion of the brain is associated with the coordination of movement, posture and balance, and cardiac, respiratory, and vasomotor functions.

The Limbic System

The limbic system includes the thalamus, hypothalamus, amygdala, and hippocampus. It is responsible for processing emotion and storing and retrieving memory.

The Thalamus

The thalamus is a large, paired, egg-shaped structure containing clusters of nuclei (gray matter); it is responsible for sensory and motor functions. Sensory information enters the thalamus, which relays the information to the overlying cerebral cortex.

The Hypothalamus

The hypothalamus is located ventral to the thalamus and is responsible for regulating emotion, thirst, hunger, circadian rhythms, the autonomic nervous system, and the pituitary gland.

The Amygdala

The amygdala is located in the temporal lobe just beneath the surface of the hippocampus and is associated with memory, emotion, and fear.

The Hippocampus

The hippocampus is that portion of the cerebral hemisphere in the basal medial part of the temporal lobe. It is responsible for learning and memory. It is also responsible for converting short-term memory to more permanent memory and for recalling spatial relationships.

The Brain Stem

The brain stem is located underneath the limbic system. It's responsible for regulating breathing, heartbeat, and blood pressure. The main constituents of the brain stem are the midbrain, pons, medulla, and the pyramidal and extrapyramidal systems.

The Midbrain

The midbrain, also called the mesencephalon, is located between the forebrain and the hindbrain (pons and medulla) and includes the tectum and the tegmentum. The midbrain participates in regulating motor functions, eye movements, pupil dilation, and hearing. The midbrain also contains the crus cerebri, which is made up of nerve fibers. These nerve fibers connect the cerebral hemispheres to the cerebellum and substantia nigra. The substantia nigra neurons are pigmented and consist of two parts, the pars reticulate and the pars compacta. Nerve cells of the pars compacta contain dark pigments (melanin granules). These neurons synthesize dopamine and project to either the caudate nucleus or the putamen. Both the caudate nucleus and the putamen are part of the basal ganglia, which regulate movement and coordination. The striatum part of the brain consists of the globus pallidus, the substantia nigra, and the basal ganglia.

The Pons

The pons (metencephalon) is located below the posterior portion of the cerebrum and above the medulla oblongata. It regulates arousal and sleep and participates in controlling autonomic functions. It also relays sensory information between the cerebrum and the cerebellum.

The Medulla (Medulla Oblongata)

The medulla, also called the myelencephalon, is the lower portion of the brain stem and is located anterior to the cerebellum. It regulates autonomic functions and relays nerve signals between the brain and the spinal cord.

The Pyramidal and Extrapyramidal Systems

Both the pyramidal and the extrapyramidal systems represent part of the motor pathways within the brain stem. Neurons of the pyramidal system have no synapses, whereas neurons of the extrapyramidal system have synapses. Nerve fibers of the pyramidal system originate in the cerebral cortex and continue on to the thalamus and medulla oblongata. The pyramidal system regulates fine movements such as control of the jaws, lips, and aspects of the face, conscious thoughts, and movements of the hands and fingers.

The major parts of the extrapyramidal system include the red nucleus, the caudate nucleus, the putamen, the substantia nigra, the globus pallidus, and the subthalamic nuclei. The extrapyramidal system dampens erratic motions, maintains muscle tone, and allows for overall functional stability.

Other Components of the Brain

Basal Ganglia

The basal ganglia are located deep in the cerebral hemisphere. They consist of the caudate nucleus, the putamen, the globus pallidus, the substantia nigra, and the subthalamic nucleus. They regulate posture and emotion, such as happiness, through dopamine. They also regulate movements and their intensity.

Neurons

Neurons (nerve cells) in the brain are highly complex, specialized cells that receive information, process it, and then send it in the form of electrical impulses through synapses to other neurons. (Synapses con-

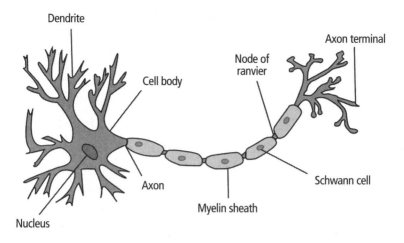

Figure 1.2. A typical neuron

nect a neuron to other neurons.) A diagrammatic representation of a neuron is provided in figure 1.2. The estimation of the number of neurons in the brain varies from study to study, with one study estimating that the human brain contains about 100 billion neurons and about 100 trillion synapses (Williams and Herrup 1988). Approximately 3 to 5 percent of neurons are lost from the brain every decade after the age of thirty-five. Therefore, it's possible that older individuals may have fewer neurons than the aforementioned estimated 100 billion neurons.

A neuron consists of the cell body (also called soma), dendrites, and an axon. The cell body contains a nucleus, mitochondria, Golgi bodies, and lysosomes, as well as smooth and rough endoplasmic reticulum. Dendrites are filamentous structures that extend away from the cell body. They branch into several processes that become thinner the farther they extend. An axon is also a filamentous structure that extends itself from the cell body at a swelling called the axon hillock, which branches away from the soma. As it extends farther it undergoes further branching at the axonal terminal. These branches, through synapses, can communicate with more than one neuron at a time.

The soma can have numerous dendrites but only one axon. The

axons of presynaptic neurons contain mitochondria and microtubules. The microtubules help to transport neurotransmitters from the cytoplasm to the tip of the axon, where they're stored in very small vesicles. Incoming synaptic signals from other neurons are received by the dendrites; the outgoing signals are sent through the axons.

Presynaptic neurons are those that transmit signals to different neurons through the axon and its synapses. The neurons that receive these signals are called postsynaptic neurons. Axon terminals contain neurotransmitters that are released at the postsynaptic neurons.

There are three major specialized neurons: sensory neurons, motor neurons, and interneurons. Sensory neurons respond to touch, sound, light, and many other stimuli. They affect the cells of sensory organs and then send signals to the brain and the spinal cord. Motor neurons receive signals from the brain and the spinal cord, cause muscle contractions, and affect glands. Interneurons connect neurons to other neurons within the same regions of the brain.

Other neurons include cholinergic neurons, dopaminergic neurons, glutamatergic neurons, GABAergic neurons, and serotonergic neurons. They are described below.

Cholinergic neurons: Cholinergic neurons are primarily located in the basal forebrain, striatum, and cerebral cortex. Each neuron contains an enzyme choline acetyltransferase, which makes the neurotransmitter acetylcholine from choline. Acetylcholine is degraded by another enzyme called acetylcholinesterase. Acetylcholine is stored in small vesicles in the nerve endings. An elevation of extracellular calcium causes the release of acetylcholine from the vesicles. The action of this neurotransmitter is mediated through nicotinic receptors and muscarinic receptors. Cholinergic neurons are the primary source of acetylcholine for the cerebral cortex; acetylcholine regulates memory and learning ability.

Dopaminergic neurons: Dopamine belongs to the group of catecholamines. It is degraded by the enzyme catechol-O-methyltransferase (COMT). Neurons that produce dopamine (dopaminergic neurons) are also referred to as dopamine (DA) neurons. Dopaminergic neurons make a neurotransmitter dopamine (3,4-dihydroxyphenethylamine) from L-dopa (L-3,4-dihydroxyphenylalanine) with the help of the enzyme DOPA decarboxylase. L-dopa is made from the amino acid tyrosine by the enzyme tyrosine hydroxylase. Dopamine neurons are primarily located in the substantia nigra pars compacta, a part of the basal ganglia present in the midbrain. This area of the brain also contains melanin granules and a high level of iron (Chinta and Andersen 2005). The presence of melanin granules and iron exposes dopamine neurons to increased levels of free radicals.

The ventral tegmental area of the midbrain also contains dopamine neurons, which send their projections to the striatum, globus pallidus, and subthalamic nucleus. Although the number of dopamine neurons is relatively less, they regulate several functions, including voluntary movement, mood reward addiction, stress, motivation, arousal, and sexual gratification. The action of dopamine is mediated via dopamine receptors D1-5. Dopamine is converted to norepinephrine by the enzyme dopamine B-carboxylase, and norepinephrine is converted to epinephrine by the enzyme phenylethanolamine-N-methyltransferase. Catecholamines (dopamine, norepinephrine, and epinephrine) are degraded by the enzyme COMT and/or monoamine oxidase.

Glutamatergic neurons: Neurons producing glutamate are called glutamatergic neurons. Glutamate is considered one of the most important neurotransmitters for proper brain functioning. As mentioned earlier it is considered excitatory because it causes hyperactivity and kills neurons by excitotoxicity. Excitotoxicity refers to the ability of glutamate to kill neurons by producing prolonged excitatory synaptic transmission. Glutamate mediates its actions through its receptors N-methyl-D-aspartate (NMDA), a-amino-3-hydroxy-5-methyl-4-isoxazolepropionic acid (AMPA), kianate, and G-protein coupled glutamate receptors (mGLuR1).

Glutamate is a nonessential amino acid that does not cross the blood-brain barrier. It is made in the neurons from glutamine that is present in the synaptic terminal. Glutamine is released from glial cells and accumulates in the presynaptic terminal where it is converted to glutamate by the mitochondrial enzyme glutaminase. Glutamate is stored in very small vesicles and is released from these vesicles by the glutamate transporters present in glial cells and presynaptic terminals. Glutamate is converted back to glutamine by the enzyme glutamine synthetase, which is present in glial cells. Glutamine is then transported from the glial cells to presynaptic nerve terminals.

More than half of the brain synapses release glutamate. Following brain injury, glutamate is released and accumulates in the extracellular space of the brain. This is responsible for the neurodegeneration that is commonly found in some neurodegenerative diseases. An increase in the extracellular levels of glutamate in the brain is associated with some neurological conditions, such as concussive injury, traumatic brain injury, post-traumatic stress disorder (PTSD), and Huntington's disease.

GABAergic neurons: Neurons producing gamma-aminobutyric acid (GABA) are called GABAergic neurons. As opposed to the excitatory function of glutamate, GABA exhibits inhibitory transmission and thereby balances the effect of glutamate on the neurons. It's been estimated that about 25 percent of neurons in the cortex use GABA (Tamminga et al. 2004). Like glutamate, GABA does not cross the blood-brain barrier. It is made in the neuron from glutamate by the enzyme L-glutamic acid decarboxylase and converted back to glutamate by a metabolic process called GABA shunt. The first step in the GABA shunt is to convert α-ketoglutarate into L-glutamic acid by the enzyme GABA α-oxoglutarate transaminase. Glutamic acid decarboxylase (GAD) converts glutamic acid into GABA.

Like glutamate, GABA is a nonessential amino acid. It mediates its action through GABA receptors (GABAa and GABAb). GABAa receptors regulate rapid mood changes as well as fear and anxiety.

These receptors are the target for sedative drugs such as alcohol, benzodiazepines, and barbiturates. GABAb receptors regulate memory and depressed moods and pain. Stimulation of this receptor can reduce the release of dopamine that would inhibit the reward response induced by external agents such as recreational drugs.

Purkinje neurons: Purkinje neurons are the largest neurons; they belong to the class of GABA neurons that are located in the cortex of the cerebellum. They can have more than a thousand dendritic branches. One Purkinje neuron can make connections with several neurons. These neurons possess a bidirectional signaling axis, which produces inhibitory as well as excitatory interneurons that play an important role in motor learning and general learning ability (Fleming et al. 2013).

Serotonergic neurons: Neurons producing serotonin (5-HT) are called serotonergic neurons. Serotonergic neurons are located in the raphe nuclei of the midbrain, pons, and medulla; they also accumulate in the synaptic clefts. The levels of serotonin in the synaptic cleft depend on the synthesis as well as the reuptake of serotonin. Serotonin neurons send projections to the cortex and basal ganglia.

Serotonin (5-hydroxytryptamine) is made from the amino acid tryptophan by the enzymes tryptophan hydroxylase and tryptophan decarboxylase. Serotonin does not cross the blood-brain barrier; however, L-tryptophan and its metabolite 5-hydroxytryptophan can enter the blood-brain barrier and increase the brain's level of serotonin. Serotonin mediates its action through serotonin receptors (5HT-1 and 5HT-2). It regulates mood, appetite, sleep, and, to some extent, memory and learning ability.

Glial Cells

Glial cells are totally different from nerve cells. Characterized by the presence of glial fibrillary acidic protein (GFAP), which is specific to them, they're considered supporting cells for the development, survival, and synaptic functions of neurons. They also help in the repair processes after an injury to the brain. Like neurons, they don't divide in the adult brain; but unlike neurons, they rapidly divide in response to brain injury. They do not have axons or elaborate neurites. The number of glial cells in the brain is much higher than the number of nerve cells. Indeed, the glial cells' main role is to support the nerve cells and to ensure their proper functioning. (The term *glial* is derived from the Greek word for "glue.") There are three types of glial cells in mature human brains: astrocytes, oligodendrocytes, and microglia.

Astrocytes: Astrocytes have small cytoplasmic processes that give an appearance of stars. They remove excess neurotransmitters released from nerve terminals and thereby regulate synaptic transmission. These cells also help to maintain concentrations of calcium and potassium in the brain.

Oligodendrocytes: Oligodendrocytes produce myelin, which wraps around the axons of neurons. The myelin sheath of oligodendrocytes forms electrical insulation around the nerve fibers and thereby facilitates rapid transmission of electrical signals in the brain.

Microglia: Microglia cells are smaller in size and are considered immune cells of the brain. In response to cellular injury the microglia migrate to the site of injury to help in the healing processes. These cells also produce pro-inflammatory cytokines that can damage neurons if the injury persists.

Growth Factors

Brains produce growth factors, which include nerve growth factor (NGF), brain-derived neurotrophic factor (BDNF), and glial cell–derived neurotrophic factor (GDNF). These growth factors are important in the development, survival, and regeneration of neurons following an injury. Both astrocytes and embryonic neurons from the mouse brain produce nerve growth factor in culture. The levels of nerve growth factor were higher in the growth phase than in the nongrowth phase. Unlike astrocytes, embryonic neurons continue to produce nerve growth factor during the nongrowth phase (Houlgatte et al. 1989).

It has been demonstrated that the presence of both glial cell–derived neurotrophic factor and brain-derived neurotrophic factor is required for the survival of certain neurons, including dopamine neurons (Erickson, Brosenitsch, and Katz 2001).

Brain-derived neurotrophic factors act via their respective receptors. In a clinical study of 91 teenagers, it was demonstrated that serum levels of brain-derived neurotrophic factor increased after exercise and improved cognitive function (Lee et al. 2014). The level of basic fibroblastic growth factor (bFGF) increases in glioma cells. It has been demonstrated that insertion of basic fibroblastic growth factor into astrocytes causes a migration and proliferation of cells without tumor formation (Holland and Varmus 1998).

This observation suggests that increased levels of basic fibroblastic growth factor are not related to cancer formation in glial cells. An elevation of basic fibroblastic growth factor may be a signal for the astrocytes to divide.

Neurotransmitters

Neurotransmitters are chemicals produced in the neurons and are located primarily at the synapses. They carry signals from one neuron to another; these signals may be inhibitory or excitatory. Neurotransmitters are released in response to a specific stimulus; all have different functions. Electrical charges from the cytoplasm of the neurons release neurotransmitters and send them across the synapse. They travel through the gap junction to bind with the receptors specific to a particular neurotransmitter located on the surface of postsynaptic neurons.

Synapses

A synapse is the junction between two neurons (presynaptic neurons and postsynaptic neurons). The gap between two neurons is about 0.02 microns.

Processes of the Brain

Conduction of Signals

To communicate neurons send electrical signals (action potential) to other neurons through the axons. This process of sending electrical signals is called conduction. An electrical signal is formed when ions, which are electrically charged particles, move across the neuronal membrane. The movement of ions takes place through ion channels that can open or close in the presence of neurotransmitters. The neuronal membrane is normally at rest (in a polarized state). The influx and outflux of ions through ion channels during neurotransmission depolarizes the target neuron. When this depolarization reaches a point of no return (threshold), a large electrical signal is generated. This electrical signal propagates along the axon until it reaches the axon terminal, where the conduction of the electrical signal ends. The neuron then sends its output to other neurons.

Synaptic Transmission (Neurotransmission)

Synaptic transmission between neurons occurs by the movement of an electric or chemical signal across a synapse. At the electrical synapse the electrical signals are considered output, whereas at the chemical synapse neurotransmitters are considered output. At the electrical synapses two neurons are physically connected to each other through the gap junction that we mentioned earlier. The gap junction allows changes in the electrical signal of one neuron to affect the other. Chemical synaptic neurotransmission occurs at the chemical synapse. In this type of transmission the presynaptic neurons and the postsynaptic neurons are separated by the synaptic cleft. The synaptic cleft allows signals coming from one neuron to pass to another neuron.

CONCLUDING REMARKS

The human brain is the body's most complex organ about which much is still unknown. It's composed of approximately 100 billion neurons and 100 trillion synapses that extend over three areas: the forebrain, midbrain, and hindbrain. Parts of the brain include the cerebrum, the cerebellum, the limbic system, and the brain stem. Four cavities filled with cerebrospinal fluid are also part of the brain.

Brain cells include the neurons mentioned above as well as glial cells. Neurons, both presynaptic and postsynaptic, hold and transmit information via the synapses in a process known as conduction. There are many different types of brain neurons; each type has a different function. Chemicals that transport signals from neuron to neuron, called neurotransmitters, are also part of the picture. Glial cells support the neurons and help to heal the brain in the case of brain injury. Substances called growth factors are produced by the brain and help neurons to recover following brain injury.

Now that we have discussed the components of the brain, its structure, and how it functions, let's turn our attention to the overall functioning of the human body in terms of how it relates to different types of stress, infection, and injury and how the immune system attempts to protect it in the face of these stressors.

2 Oxidative Stress, Inflammation, and the Immune System

This chapter describes oxidative stress caused by free radicals, types and sources of free radicals, inflammation, and the immune system briefly and in general terms.* These issues are huge and complex, but herein we have attempted to describe them simply so that they may be easily grasped. A basic understanding of these biological processes and agents is essential for developing strategies for prevention and improved management of the debilitating neurodegenerative diseases such as Parkinson's disease and Huntington's disease.

WHAT IS OXIDATIVE STRESS?

Oxidative stress is a process that occurs when free radicals overwhelm the protective antioxidant systems of the body. What are free radicals? They are atoms, molecules, or ions with unpaired electrons—

---

*Some of the references and books that have been used to prepare this chapter are Cotran 1999; Ryter 1985; Langermans, Hazenbos, and van Furth 1994; Holtmeier and Kabelitz 2005; Sproul et al. 2000; Kehry and Hodgkin 1994; Asmus 1994; Vaillancourt et al. 2008; Pryor 1994; and Kehrer 1994.

derived from either oxygen or nitrogen—which makes them highly reactive. However, although they can damage cells, they also play an important role in the regulation of certain biochemical processes and gene expressions necessary for our survival. In 1900 the first organic free radical, triphenylmethyl radical, was identified by Moses Gomberg of the University of Michigan. Free radicals are symbolized by a dot "•".

The half-lives of various free radicals vary from 10^{-9} seconds to days. This means most are quickly destroyed after causing damage. For example, the half-life of hydroxyl free radicals is 10^{-9} seconds, superoxide anion 10^{-5} seconds, lipid peroxyl free radical 7 seconds, semiquinone free radical days, nitric oxide about 1 second, and hydrogen peroxide minutes. The half-lives of some organic free radicals are several days.

TYPES OF FREE RADICALS

There are several different types of free radicals derived from oxygen and nitrogen that are generated in the body. The oxygen-derived free radicals include hydroxyl radical (OH•), peroxyl radical (ROO•), alkoxyl radical (RO•), phenoxyl and semiquinone radicals (ArO•, HO-Ar-O•), and superoxide radical ($O^{•-}_2$). The nitrogen-derived free radicals include, NO, •ONOO⁻ (peroxynitrite), and •NO_2.

SOURCES OF FREE RADICALS

Normally free radicals are generated in the body during the use of oxygen in the metabolism of certain compounds. Mitochondria, which are elongated membranous structures present in all cells in varying numbers, use oxygen to produce energy. During the process of generating energy, superoxide anions, hydroxyl radicals, and hydrogen peroxide are produced as by-products. It is estimated that about 2 percent of the oxygen consumed by the mitochondria remains partially used, and this unused oxygen leaks out of the mitochondria to make approximately 20 billion molecules of superoxide anions and hydrogen peroxide per cell per day.

During bacterial or viral infection, phagocytic cells are activated, generating high levels of nitric oxide superoxide anions and hydrogen peroxide within the infected cells in order to kill infective agents. Excessive production of free radicals by phagocytes can also damage normal cells, thereby increasing the risk of acute and/or chronic disease.

During the oxidative metabolism of fatty acids and other molecules in the body, free radicals are produced. Certain habits such as tobacco smoking, and the presence of some trace minerals such as free iron, copper, and manganese, can also increase the rate of production of free radicals. Thus is the human body exposed daily to different types and varying levels of free radicals.

OXIDATION AND REDUCTION PROCESSES

To more fully understand the role that free radicals play, it's beneficial to grasp the relationship between the processes of oxidation and reduction that are constantly taking place in the body.

Oxidation is a process by which an atom or a molecule gains oxygen, loses hydrogen, or loses an electron. For example, carbon gains oxygen during oxidation and becomes carbon dioxide. A superoxide radical loses an electron during the oxidation process and becomes oxygen. Thus, an *oxidizing agent* is an atom or molecule that changes another chemical by adding oxygen to it or by removing an electron or hydrogen from it. Examples of oxidizing agents include free radicals, X-rays, and ozone.

Other oxidizing agents formed in the body include peroxynitrite, hydrogen peroxide, and lipid peroxide, all of which are very damaging to the cells. Many other radical species can be formed by biological reactions. These include phenolic and other aromatic compounds that are formed during metabolism of xenobiotic agents (agents that are foreign to the body).

Reduction is a process by which an atom or molecule loses oxygen, gains hydrogen, or gains an electron. For example, carbon dioxide loses oxygen and becomes carbon monoxide, carbon gains hydrogen and becomes methane, and oxygen gains an electron and becomes a superoxide anion. Thus, a *reducing agent* is an atom or molecule that changes another chemical by removing oxygen from it or by adding an electron or hydrogen to it.

All antioxidants may be considered reducing agents. Increased reduction processes over oxidation processes maintain cells in a healthy state; however, increased oxidation processes over reduction processes can lead to cellular injury and eventually to chronic neurodegenerative diseases.

As we have learned, oxidative stress occurs when the generation of reactive oxygen species exceeds the antioxidant defense system's ability to neutralize them. Similarly, nitrosylative stress occurs when the generation of reactive nitrogen species exceeds the antioxidant defense system's ability to neutralize them. A chronic increase in oxidative and nitrosylative stress has been implicated in the initiation and progression of most chronic diseases in humans. However, short-term increased oxidative stress such as is seen during viral or bacterial infection may be important in killing invading organisms (although it can also damage normal tissue). Free radicals can damage DNA (deoxyribonucleic acid), RNA (ribonucleic acid), proteins, carbohydrates, and membranes.

The Formation of Free Radicals Derived
from Oxygen and Nitrogen

The formative process of some reactive oxygen species (ROS: free radicals derived from oxygen) is described below.

When molecular oxygen (O_2) acquires an electron, the superoxide anion ($O_2^{•-}$) is formed:

$$O_2 + e^- = O_2^{•-}$$

Superoxide dismutase (SOD) and H^+ can react with $O_2^{•-}$ to form hydrogen peroxide (H_2O_2):

$$2O_2^{•-} + 2H^+ \text{ plus SOD} \rightarrow H_2O_2 + O_2$$
$$O_2^{•-} + H^+ \rightarrow HO_2^{•} \text{ (hydroperoxy radical)}$$
$$2HO_2^{•} \rightarrow H_2O_2 + O_2$$

Ferric and ferrous forms of iron can react with superoxide anion and hydrogen peroxide to produce molecular oxygen (O_2) and hydroxyl radicals ($OH^{•}$), respectively:

$$Fe^{3+} + O_2^{•-} \rightarrow Fe^{2+} + O_2$$
$$Fe_2^+ + H_2O_2 \rightarrow Fe^{3+} + OH^{•} + OH^- \text{ (Fenton reaction)}$$

Hydroxyl radicals can also be formed from superoxide anion by the Haber-Weiss reaction:

$$O_2^{•-} + H_2O_2 \rightarrow O_2 + OH^- + OH^{•}$$

Both the Fenton and Haber-Weiss reactions require a transition metal such as copper or iron. Among ROS, $OH^{•}$ is the most damaging free radical and is very short-lived.

Hydroxyl radicals are very reactive with a variety of organic compounds, leading to the production of more radical compounds:

$$RH \text{ (organic compound)} + OH^{•} \rightarrow R^{•} \text{ (organic radical)} + H_2O$$
$$R^{•} + O_2 \rightarrow RO_2^{•} \text{ (peroxyl radical)}$$

For example, the DNA radical can be generated by reaction with a hydroxyl radical, and this can lead to a break in the DNA strand.

Catalase detoxifies hydrogen peroxide to form water and molecular oxygen:

$$H_2O_2 + catalase \rightarrow H_2O \text{ and } O_2$$

Reactive nitrogen species (RNS: free radicals derived from nitrogen) are represented by nitric oxide ($NO^{\bullet}$). NO is synthesized by the enzyme nitric oxide synthase from L-arginine. $NO^{\bullet}$ can combine with superoxide anion to form peroxynitrite, a powerful oxidant.

$$NO^{\bullet} + O_2^{\bullet -} \rightarrow ONOO^- \text{ (peroxynitrite)}$$

When protonated (likely at physiological pH), peroxynitrite spontaneously decomposes to reactive nitric dioxide and hydroxyl radicals:

$$ONOO^- + H^+ \rightarrow {}^{\bullet}NO_2 + OH^{\bullet}$$

Superoxide dismutase (SOD) can also enhance the peroxynitrite-mediated nitration of tyrosine residues on critical proteins, presumably via species similar to the nitronium cation (NO_2^+):

$$ONOO^- \text{ plus SOD} \rightarrow NO_2^+ \rightarrow \text{Nitration of tyrosine}$$

WHAT IS INFLAMMATION?

Inflammation in Latin is referred to as *inflammare,* which means "setting on fire." Inflammation is a complex biological response initiated by the immune system. It removes infective agents such as bacteria and viruses and helps to repair tissue damage caused by ionizing radiation, toxic chemicals, and/or traumatic injuries to the body. Immune cells in the peripheral blood, such as neutrophils and macrophages, participate in inflammatory reactions. In the brain, microglia are considered to be the inflammatory cells.

Primary features of inflammation at the affected site include redness, swelling, and warmth when touched, in addition to varying degrees of pain. These characteristics of inflammation were first recognized by the renowned Roman medical scholar Aulus Cornelius Celsus (circa 25 BCE to 50 CE).

The injured or infected cells release eicosanoids and cytokines. Growth factors and cytotoxic factors are also released. These cytokines and other chemicals recruit immune cells (white blood cells—leukocytes, macrophages, monocytes, lymphocytes, and plasma cells) to the site of infection to eliminate invading, harmful organisms or to promote the healing of injured tissue (Martin and Leibovich 2005).

As the body removes the injurious infective microorganisms as well as initiates the healing process, the injured tissue is replaced by the regeneration of native parenchymal cells (original cell type), by filling of the injured site with fibroblastic tissue (scarring), or most commonly by a combination of both processes. During inflammation toxic chemicals that may damage cells are also released.

TYPES OF INFLAMMATION

Inflammation is divided into two categories: acute and chronic. Acute inflammation occurs following cellular injury or infection with microorganisms. The period of acute inflammation is relatively short, lasting from a few minutes to a few days. The main features of acute inflammation are edema (accumulation of exudation of fluid and plasma in extracellular spaces) and the migration of leukocytes, primarily neutrophils, to the site of injury.

Chronic inflammation is a second form of inflammation. It occurs following persistent cellular injury or infection. The period of chronic inflammation is relatively long and can last as long as the injury or infection exists. The main features of chronic inflammation are the presence of lymphocytes and macrophages and the proliferation of blood vessels, fibrosis, and tissue necrosis.

Let's examine both types of inflammation in further detail below.

Acute Inflammation

Acute inflammation causes marked alterations in blood vessels, which allow plasma protein and leukocytes to leave the body's primary circulation pathways. Subsequently, the leukocytes migrate to the site of injury by a process called chemotaxis. Leukocytes engulf pathogenic organisms by phagocytosis and then kill them by generating bursts of reactive oxygen species (ROS) and other toxic substances. They can also engulf cellular debris and foreign antigens by a similar process and then degrade them with lysosomal proteolytic enzymes.

Leukocytes, however, may release excessive amounts of ROS, pro-inflammatory cytokines, prostaglandins, adhesion molecules, and complement proteins and thus can damage normal tissue. An acute inflammatory reaction is tightly regulated and turned off soon after the injured sites are healed or the invading microbes removed.

Acute inflammation is an essential process for the removal of pathogens (harmful organisms) and cellular debris from the damaged site, thus allowing healing to occur. However, it is effective only when the injurious stimuli or tissue damage is relatively mild. If the tissue damage is extensive, or the levels of infective organisms are high, acute inflammatory reactions are not turned off. Consequently, the toxic products of these reactions can enhance the rate of damage, which may cause organ failure and eventually even death.

Chronic Inflammation

Persistent low-grade cellular injury or exposure to exogenous agents such as particulate silica or infection can initiate chronic inflammation. Chronic inflammation is often associated with most human neurodegenerative conditions and diseases.

In contrast to acute inflammation, which is characterized by vascular changes, edema, and primarily neutrophil infiltration, chronic inflammation is characterized by the presence of mononuclear cells, which include macrophages, lymphocytes, and plasma cells. In the brain microglia cells become activated and migrate to the site of injury. During chronic inflammation the presence of angiogenesis and fibrosis can be observed at the site of injury.

Although the acute inflammatory responses may produce pro-inflammatory cytokines, ROS, prostaglandins, adhesion molecules, and complements, the chronic inflammatory processes more typically do so. Therefore they are more relevant to neurodegenerative diseases when compared to acute inflammatory reactions. As we have learned, the release of these agents is tightly regulated and is mitigated when the invading pathogenic (harmful) organisms are killed or the injured tissues are healed. In chronic inflammation, on the other hand, the inflammatory response to chronic cellular injury or chronic infection is not turned off.

PRODUCTS OF INFLAMMATORY REACTIONS

As we know, during inflammation several highly reactive agents are released. They include cytokines, complement proteins, arachidonic acid (AA) metabolites, ROS, and endothelial/leukocyte adhesion molecules. They are briefly described below.

Cytokines

Cytokines are proteins released during both acute and chronic inflammation. They are produced by many cell types, primarily by activated lymphocytes and macrophages but also by endothelium, epithelium, and connective tissue cells. In the brain they are produced primarily by microglia cells and some by neurons. Pro-inflammatory cytokines include interleukin-6 (IL-6), IL-17, IL-18, IL-23, and tumor necrosis factor-alpha (TNF-alpha) that are toxic to the cells. Anti-inflammatory cytokines include IL-1, IL-4, IL-10, IL-11, and IL-13, which help in the repair at the site of injury.

If the tissue damage is severe, the pro-inflammatory cytokines may overcome the repair function of the anti-inflammatory cytokines and participate in the progression of damage. Some pro-inflammatory cytokines such as IL-6 can also act as a neurotrophic factor. In this it functions as a pro-inflammatory cytokine during the acute phase of injury and as a neurotrophic factor between the subacute and chronic phase of injury.

Cytokines play an important role in modulating the function of many other cell types. They are multifunctional, and individual cytokines may have both positive and negative regulatory actions. Cytokines mediate their action by binding to specific receptors on target cells. These receptors are regulated by exogenous and endogenous signals. Cytokines that regulate lymphocyte activation, growth, and differentiation include interleukin-2 (IL-2) and IL-4 (favors growth), as well as IL-10 and transforming growth factor-beta (TGF-beta), which are negative regulators of immune responses.

Cytokines involved with natural immunity include tumor necrosis factor-alpha (TNF-alpha), IL-1Beta, type I interferon (IFN-alpha and IFN-beta), and IL-6. Cytokines that activate inflammatory cells such as macrophages include IFN-gamma, TNF-alpha, TNF-beta, IL-5, IL-10, and IL-12. Cytokines that stimulate hematopoiesis (growth and differentiation of immature leukocytes) include IL-3, IL-7, c-kit ligand, granulocyte-macrophage colony-stimulating factor (GM-CSF), macrophage colony-stimulating factor (M-CSF), granulocyte CSF, and stem cell factor.

Chemokines are also cytokines that stimulate leukocyte movement and direct them to the site of injury during inflammation. Many classical growth factors may also act as cytokines, and, conversely, many cytokines exhibit activities of growth factors.

Complement Proteins

During inflammation twenty complement proteins, including their cleavage (degradation) products, are released into the plasma, and when activated they can cause cell lysis (death). They can also exhibit proteolytic activity. They participate in both innate and adaptive immunity for protection against pathogenic organisms; however, they are considered major humoral components of the innate immune response (Rus, Cudrici, and Niculescu 2005). Complement proteins participate in killing pathogenic microorganisms with the antibodies through complex mechanisms. Complement proteins are numbered C1 through C9. All of them have complex mechanisms of action on cells. Some complement proteins are also neurotoxic.

Arachidonic Acid (AA) Metabolites

Arachidonic acid is a 20-carbon fatty acid that is derived from dietary sources or is formed from the essential fatty acid linoleic acid. During inflammation, AA metabolites, also called eicosanoids, are released. These eicosanoids have diverse biological actions, depending upon the cell type, and they are synthesized by two major classes of enzymes: cyclooxygenase (COX) for the synthesis of prostaglandins and thromboxanes, and lipooxygenase for the synthesis of leukotrienes and lipoxins. There are two isoforms of cyclooxygenase: COX-1 and COX-2.

ROS

ROS consists of free radicals derived from the oxygen.

Endothelial/Leukocyte Adhesion Molecules

The immunoglobulin family of molecules includes two endothelial adhesion molecules: intracellular adhesion molecule-1 (ICAM-1) and vascular adhesion molecule-1 (VCAM-1). These adhesion molecules bind with leukocyte receptor integrins. They are induced by IL-1 and TNF-alpha. Both ICAM-1 and VCAM-1 are released during inflammatory reactions and have diverse mechanisms of action on cells.

Leukocytes include the phagocytes (primarily macrophages and neutrophils) and dendritic cells, mast cells, eosinophils, basophils, and natural killer cells. These cells identify and kill harmful microorganisms by phagocytosis. Phagocytosis is an important feature of cellular innate immunity. Neutrophils and macrophages are the most active in phagocytosis following infection with pathogenic microorganisms. These cells engulf pathogens that are trapped in an intracellular vesicle called phago-somes, which fuse with lysosomes to form phagolysosomes. The harmful organisms are killed by proteolytic enzymes (enzymes that can digest) of the lysosomes aided by bursts of ROS released by the phagocytes. Natural killer cells can kill tumor cells or cells infected with viruses.

WHAT IS THE IMMUNE SYSTEM?

The immune system is a network of cells, tissues, and organs that works together in a highly coordinated manner to defend the body against for-eign pathogenic organisms or antigenic molecules or particles. It plays an important role in defense against invading pathogenic (harmful) organisms; therefore, it's essential for survival. Under certain conditions the immune system can produce toxic chemicals that play an impor-tant role in the initiation and progression of chronic neurodegenerative diseases as well as causing autoimmune diseases.

The immune system is highly complex and tightly regulated. On one hand, it defends the body against foreign pathogenic microorganisms and antigenic molecules or particles. On the other hand, it has the ability to produce toxic chemicals such as ROS, pro-inflammatory cytokines, com-plement proteins, adhesion molecules, and prostaglandins, all of which are toxic to the tissues. These toxic chemicals may increase the risk of chronic conditions, including neurodegenerative conditions. Furthermore, the presence of endogenous antigens can initiate an immune response that damages the body's own tissue such as is seen in rheumatoid arthritis.

Once the immune system has been exposed to an antigen and suc-cessfully removes it, it stores the recognition factor of this antigen in its memory. Thus, during the lifetime of an individual, the immune system stores recognition factors of millions of different antigens and protects the body from these antigens all the time. This process of exposure to an antigen and successfully removing it is generally referred to as acquired immunity, which is the basis of vaccination.

The organs of the immune system are located throughout the body. They are lymphoid organs that contain lymphocytes and bone marrow that contain all types of blood cells, including lymphocytes. Thymus-derived lymphocytes are referred to as T-lymphocytes (T-cells). In the blood T-cells represent about 60 to 70 percent of peripheral lymphocytes. Lymphocytes derived from bone marrow are referred to as B-lymphocytes (B-cells). They constitute about 10 to 20 percent of peripheral lymphocytes in the blood. B-cells mature to plasma cells that secrete specific antibodies in response to a particular antigen.

Macrophages are derived from monocytes of bone marrow and are a part of the mononuclear phagocyte system. They exhibit phagocytic activity, which is essential for removing harmful organisms from the body. A specialized form of cells with numerous fine dendritic cytoplasmic processes, called dendritic cells, does not exhibit phagocytic activity. They play an important role in presenting antigen to T-cells. Natural killer (NK) cells represent about 10 to 15 percent of the peripheral blood lymphocytes and lack T-cell receptors. They can kill tumor cells.

The major components of the immune system are innate immunity and adaptive immunity. The innate immune defenses are nonspecific, but it is the dominant system of host defense (Litman, Cannon, and Dishaw 2005). The innate immune response is activated when microorganisms are identified by pattern of recognition receptors or when damaged cells send signals to the immune system for a defensive response (Medzhitov 2007; Matzinger 2002). The innate immune responses do not confer long-lasting immunity against pathogenic organisms. The innate immune system responds to infection by inducing inflammation, releasing complement proteins, and recruiting leukocytes.

INNATE IMMUNITY

The components of innate immunity include inflammation, complement proteins, and leukocytes, all of which we have detailed earlier in this chapter. Innate immunity can activate adaptive immunity.

ADAPTIVE IMMUNITY

The adaptive response to an antigen is strong and is responsible for storing and recalling immunologic memory for recognizing and eliminating a specific antigen all the time. The lymphocytes (T-cells and B-cells) are responsible for the adaptive immune response. Both T-cells and B-cells carry receptors that recognize specific targets. T-cells can recognize only membrane-bound antigens. The cell surface of major histocompatibility complex (MHC) molecules binds peptide fragments of foreign proteins for presentation to appropriate antigen-specific T-cells. There are two major subtypes of T-cells: the killer T-cells and the helper T-cells. The killer T-cells can recognize antigens bound to Class I MHC molecules, whereas the helper cells recognize antigens bound to Class II MHC molecules. A minor subtype of T-cells is gamma-delta T-cells, which recognize intact antigens that are not bound to MHC receptors.

In contrast to the T-cells, the surface of B-cells has antibody molecules for a specific antigen. The antibody molecules recognize whole, harmful organisms and do not need any antigen-presenting mechanism for their action. Each lineage of B-cell expresses a different antibody. A B-cell first identifies pathogens (harmful microorganism) when an antibody on its surface binds to a specific foreign antigen. This antibody/antigen complex is engulfed by the B-cell, where it is converted into peptides by proteolytic enzymes. The B-cells then display on their surface antigenic peptides and Class II MHC molecules that attract matching T-helper cells that release lymphokines and activate B-cells.

The activated B-cells proliferate and differentiate to plasma cells that secrete millions of copies of the antibody that recognize this antigen. These antibodies circulate in the blood and the lymph and bind to pathogens expressing this particular antigen. These antibody/antigen-bound pathogens are destroyed by complement protein activation or by phagocytes. Antibodies can also neutralize bacterial toxins by directly binding to them. They kill bacteria or viruses by interfering with their receptors, which are used to infect cells.

CONCLUDING REMARKS

Free radicals are products of a biological process that occurs naturally as a result of the body's constant use of oxygen. For the past half a century its significance as a contributory factor to the aging process has become more widely recognized, as has the understanding that it exists in part as an imbalance of our gene expression. Oxidative stress occurs when there is an excessive production of free radicals in the body; these may be derived from oxygen or from nitrogen. An excessive production of free radicals may pave the way for disease, given that an overabundance of toxic free radicals are capable of damaging the body's cells and tissues unless they can be neutralized by the body's defensive systems.

These defensive systems include the processes of the antioxidant defense system, anti-inflammation products, and the immune system itself. Antioxidants destroy free radicals. When one is injured or has an infection, the immune system immediately initiates actions to set a healing cascade in place. When this happens, white blood cells and anti-inflammatory compounds are called to the site of infection or injury to repair the damage. Once these agents have completed their work and the healing process is complete, the healing agents recede. However, if the immune system is compromised, or the injury overwhelms the immune system, the cellular damage may persist, and a state of chronic inflammation may ensue.

The initiation and progression of most chronic neurodegenerative diseases are characterized by increased oxidative stress, chronic inflammation, and glutamate release. If these biological events can be adequately controlled and managed, one reduces the risk of developing the debilitating neurological conditions that are the subjects of this book.

3 Properties and Functions of Vitamins and Antioxidant Systems

This chapter presents a broad overview of antioxidants and details many of their qualities and characteristics. This discussion is important for a more enhanced understanding of these valuable substances and will be a useful guide for those individuals seeking a greater inclusion of them through diet and/or supplementation. Specifically, the discussion in this chapter focuses on the history, functions, sources and forms, absorption, solubility, and availability of antioxidants. It also covers other practical matters, such as how to most effectively store antioxidants in the home, whether they may be destroyed in cooking, and possible toxicity concerns.

We will end the chapter with a discussion of current controversies that exist regarding the use of antioxidants in the prevention of chronic disease.

A CLOSER LOOK AT ANTIOXIDANTS

Antioxidants are chemical micronutrients that donate an electron to a free radical and convert it into a harmless molecule. They are considered to be micronutrients. But what exactly is a micronutrient? In defining micronutrients it's important to distinguish them from macronutrients. Primarily, macronutrients include fats, carbohydrates, and proteins. Micronutrients, on the other hand, include antioxidant systems represented by dietary and endogenous antioxidant chemicals; polyphenolic compounds derived from fruits, vegetables, and plants; the mineral selenium; and B vitamins as well as vitamin D.

Although *all* micronutrients are essential for human survival and growth, antioxidants have enjoyed a special focus in this regard. They have been the subject of extensive laboratory research and clinical studies because of their potential importance in reducing oxidative stress and inflammation, which could decrease the risk of chronic disease.

Polyphenolic compounds derived from herbs also exhibit antioxidant and anti-inflammatory activities; however, they act in part by different mechanisms. Some of them reduce oxidative stress by activating the nuclear transcription factor Nrf2, which increases the levels of antioxidant enzymes by upregulating the antioxidant response element. Some dietary and endogenous antioxidants also activate Nrf2. Therefore, a combination of antioxidant chemicals and polyphenolic compounds may optimally reduce oxidative stress and inflammation.

The antioxidant defense system in humans can be divided into four groups, as follows:

Group 1 Antioxidants

These antioxidants are not made in the body but are consumed primarily through the diet. They include vitamin A, carotenoids, vitamin C, vitamin E, and selenium. They directly scavenge free radicals.

Group 2 Antioxidants

Group 2 antioxidants are made in the body and are also consumed through the diet (primarily through meat and eggs) or in the form of supplements. They include glutathione, coenzyme Q10, reduced nicotinamide adenine dinucleotide (NAD+), n-acetylcysteine (NAC), alpha-lipoic acid, and L-carnitine.

Group 3 Antioxidants

Group 3 antioxidants include antioxidants derived from fruit, vegetables, and plants. They also include polyphenolic compounds such as curcumin and resveratrol, which can be taken through the diet. However, dietary sources of these polyphenolic compounds may not provide sufficient amounts needed for the prevention of chronic neurological conditions. Thus supplementation may be necessary for optimal biological activity in the body. Both curcumin and resveratrol activate a nuclear transcriptional factor (Nrf2), which increases the levels of antioxidant enzymes through the antioxidant response element.

Group 4 Antioxidants

Another form of antioxidants are antioxidant enzymes that are made in the body. They include superoxide dismutase (SOD), catalase, and glutathione peroxidase. Superoxide dismutase requires manganese (Mn) or copper-zinc (Cu-Zn) SOD for its biological activity. Mn-SOD is present in the mitochondria, whereas Cu-Zn SOD is present in the cytoplasm. Both can destroy free radicals and hydrogen peroxide. Catalase requires iron (Fe) for its biological activity. It too destroys hydrogen peroxide in the cell. Glutathione peroxidase requires selenium for its biological activity.

THE ROLE OF ANTIOXIDANTS

Antioxidants have many valuable roles to play in safeguarding human health. Given that they're so successful in neutralizing free radicals, many people believe that this is their only function. However, in view of recent advances in antioxidant research, this belief has been proved incorrect. The actions of antioxidants on cells and tissues are varied and complex. Antioxidants and polyphenolic compounds work to:

1. Scavenge free radicals
2. Decrease markers of pro-inflammatory cytokines
3. Alter gene expression profiles
4. Alter protein kinase activity
5. Prevent the release and toxicity of excessive amounts of glutamate
6. Act as cofactors for several biological reactions
7. Induce cell differentiation and apoptosis in cancer cells
8. Induce cell differentiation in normal cells, but not apoptosis
9. Increase immune function
10. Activate Nrf2, which is essential for increasing the levels of antioxidant enzymes and phase-2-detoxyfying enzymes

HISTORY OF ANTIOXIDANTS

Vitamin A

Night blindness existed for centuries before the discovery of vitamin A. As early as 1500 BCE, Egyptians knew how to cure night blindness. Roman soldiers suffering from this condition traveled to Egypt, where they received liver extract as treatment. (Today it is well established that liver is the richest source of vitamin A.) Treating night blindness with liver extract was not employed outside of Egypt for centuries, perhaps because medical establishments in other countries during that time period did not deem it to be an acceptable treatment protocol.

In 1912, Dr. Elmer McCollum of the University of Wisconsin discovered vitamin A in butter, at which time it was named "fat-soluble A." The structure of vitamin A was determined in 1930, and it was synthesized in the laboratory in 1947.

It should be underscored that the medical establishment of that very early period, by denying the validity of vitamin A to cure night blindness, no doubt delayed the cure for blindness for centuries.

The Vitamin B Family

All of the B vitamins were discovered between 1912 and 1934. In the year 1912 the Polish biochemist Dr. Casimir Funk isolated their active substances from the rice husks of unpolished rice; these active substances prevented the disease beriberi. This disease affects many parts of the body including muscle tissue, the heart, the nervous system, and the digestive tract. Dr. Funk named the substances he discovered "vitamines," because he thought they were amines, derived from ammonia. In 1920 the *e* was dropped when it became known that not all vitamins are amines. Today there are many different vitamins in the vitamin B family.

Vitamin C

A vitamin C deficiency causes scurvy, the symptoms of which were known to Egyptians as early as 1500 BCE. In the fifth century Hippocrates described these symptoms. They include bleeding gums, hemorrhaging, and death. Native Americans had a cure for scurvy that involved drinking an extract made from the bark and needles of the pine tree, prepared like a tea. This remedy, however, remained limited to their own population for hundreds of years. Today we know that pine bark and needles are rich in vitamin C.

During the sea voyages of European explorers between the twelfth and sixteenth centuries the epidemic of scurvy among sailors forced some of them to land in Canada, where Native Americans gave them the indigenous concoction, thereby curing their illness. In 1536 the French explorer Jacques Cartier brought this formulation to France, but the medical establishment rejected it as bogus because it had originated with the Native Americans, whom they looked down upon. In 1593, Sir Richard Hawkins began recommending that his sailors eat sour oranges and lemons to reduce the risk of the disease. It would be almost another two hundred years before the British Navy began recommending that ships carry sufficient lime juice for all personnel on board. In 1928,

Albert Szent-Györgyi, a Hungarian scientist, isolated hexuronic acid from the adrenal gland. This substance was vitamin C, and in 1932 it was the first vitamin to be made in the laboratory.

It should be emphasized that the sixteenth-century medical community in France, by rejecting the use of vitamin C to treat scurvy, delayed the cure of this disease for centuries.

Carotenoids/Beta-Carotene

In 1919 carotenoid pigments were isolated from yellow plants, and in 1930 researchers found that some of the ingested carotene was converted to vitamin A. This substance is referred to as beta-carotene.

Vitamin D

Although the bone disease rickets may have existed in human populations for a long time, it wasn't until 1645 that Dr. Daniel Whistler described its symptoms. In 1922, Sir Edward Mellanby discovered vitamin D while working on a cure for rickets, which vitamin D proved to be. This vitamin was later found to require sunlight for its formation in skin cells. The chemical structure of vitamin D was determined by German scientist Dr. Adolf Windaus in 1930. Vitamin D_3 is the most active form of vitamin D. It was chemically characterized in 1936 and was initially thought to be a steroid effective in the treatment of rickets.

Vitamin E

In 1922, Dr. Herbert Evans of the University of California, Berkeley, observed that rats reared exclusively on whole milk grew normally but were not fertile. Fertility was restored when they were fed wheat germ. However, it took another fourteen years before the active substance that was responsible for restoring fertility was isolated. When this was achieved Dr. Evans named the substance tocopherol, from the Greek word meaning "to bear offspring." The added *ol* at the end signifies its chemical status as an alcohol.

Coenzyme Q10

In 1957, Dr. Fredrick Crane isolated coenzyme Q10. In 1958, Dr. Wolf, working under Dr. Karl Folkers, determined the structure of coenzyme Q10.

FUNCTIONS
OF SPECIFIC ANTIOXIDANTS

Vitamin A

In addition to destroying free radicals, vitamin A plays an important role in maintaining vision and skin health; stimulating immune function; maintaining bone metabolism; regulating gene activity, embryonic development, and reproduction; and inhibiting precancerous and cancerous cell proliferation.

Alpha-lipoic Acid

Alpha-lipoic acid is a more potent antioxidant than vitamin C or vitamin E. It's soluble in both water and lipid and thus protects cellular membranes as well as water-soluble compounds. It regenerates tissue levels of vitamin C and vitamin E and markedly elevates glutathione level in the cells. Alpha-lipoic acid acts as a cofactor for multi-enzyme dehydrogenase complexes.

Vitamin C

Vitamin C acts as an antioxidant and participates as a cofactor for the activities of some enzymes, which is essential for the formation of many vital compounds in our body. Vitamin C helps in the formation of collagen, and it also takes part in the formation of interferon, a naturally occurring antiviral agent. It regenerates oxidized vitamin E to a reduced form, which acts as an antioxidant.

Carotenoids

Beta-carotene is a precursor of vitamin A. Carotenes are known to protect against ultraviolet-light-induced damage. Beta-carotene increases the expression of the connexin gene, which codes for a gap junction protein that holds two normal cells together. (Vitamin A can't produce such an effect.) In addition, when compared to vitamins A and E, beta-carotene is a more effective destroyer of free radicals in an internal body environment that is marked by high oxygen pressure in the tissues.

Coenzyme Q10
Coenzyme Q10 is a weak antioxidant, but it recycles vitamin E. Coenzyme Q10 is essential for mitochondria to generate energy.

Vitamin D_3
Vitamin D_3 is essential for bone formation and regulates calcium and phosphorus levels in the blood. Vitamin D_3 also inhibits parathyroid hormone secretion from the parathyroid glands. It stimulates immune function by promoting phagocytosis and also exhibits antitumor activity.

Vitamin E
Vitamin E acts as an antioxidant and regulates gene expression. It also translocates certain proteins from one cellular compartment to another. Additionally, it helps to maintain skin texture, reduces scarring, and acts as an anticoagulant. Vitamin E reduces inflammation and stimulates immune function. Its derivative, vitamin E succinate, exhibits potent anticancer activities.

Glutathione
Glutathione is one of the most important antioxidants in that it protects cellular components inside the cells. It is needed for detoxification, either of certain exogenous toxins or those generated as by-products of normal metabolism. Glutathione also acts as a substrate for several enzymes. It reduces inflammation.

Melatonin

Melatonin is important in regulating circadian rhythms through its receptor. It also acts as an antioxidant and reduces inflammation. Unlike other antioxidants, the oxidation of melatonin is irreversible and thus cannot be regenerated by other antioxidants. Melatonin also stimulates immune function.

N-acetylcysteine (NAC)

N-acetylcysteine increases the glutathione levels within the cells. This function is important, because orally administered glutathione is totally destroyed in the small intestine. At high doses n-acetylcysteine binds with metals and removes them from the body.

Nicotinamide (Vitamin B₃)

Treatment with nicotinamide restored memory deficits in Alzheimer's disease transgenic mice (Green et al. 2008), attenuated glutamate-induced toxicity, and preserved cellular levels of NAD+ to support the activity of silent information regulator-1 (SIRT1) (Liu, Pitta, and Mattson 2008). Treatment with nicotinamide reduced oxidative-stress-induced mitochondrial dysfunction and increased the survival of neurons in culture. The reduced form of NAD (NADH) acts as an antioxidant and is essential for mitochondria energy.

Polyphenolic Compounds

Polyphenolic compounds exhibit antioxidant activity and reduce inflammation. They also regulate the expression of certain genes. Some polyphenolic compounds such as resveratrol and curcumin also increase the levels of antioxidant enzymes by activating a nuclear transcriptional factor, Nrf2.

SOURCES AND FORMS
OF ANTIOXIDANTS

Vitamin A

Liver from beef, pork, chicken, turkey, and fish is the richest source of vitamin A (6.5 milligrams per 100 grams of liver). Other rich sources are carrot (0.8 milligram per 100 grams), broccoli (0.8 milligram per 100 grams), sweet potato (0.7 milligram per 100 grams), kale (0.7 milligram per 100 grams), butter (0.7 milligram per 100 grams), spinach (0.5 milligram per 100 grams), and pumpkin (0.4 milligram per 100 grams). Minor sources include cantaloupe, egg, apricot, papaya, and mango (40 to 170 micrograms per 100 grams). Yellow and red fruits and vegetables are very rich sources of beta-carotene. One molecule of beta-carotene is converted to two molecules of retinol in the intestinal tract.

Vitamin A exists as retinyl palmitate or retinyl acetate that's converted into the retinol form in the body. Vitamin A exists as a retinoic acid in the cells. It has been determined that 1 IU (international unit) equals 0.3 microgram of retinol, or 0.6 microgram of beta-carotene. The activity of vitamin A is also expressed as retinol activity equivalent (RAE). One microgram of RAE corresponds to 1 microgram of retinol and 2 micrograms of beta-carotene in oil. Vitamin A, beta-carotene, and the synthetic retinoids are also available commercially.

Vitamin C

The richest source of vitamin C is fruits and vegetables, which include rose hip (2,000 milligrams per 100 grams), red pepper (2,000 milligrams per 100 grams), parsley (2,000 milligrams per 100 grams), guava (2,000 milligrams per 100 grams), kiwi fruit (2,000 milligrams per 100 grams), broccoli (2,000 milligrams per 100 grams), lychee (2,000 milligrams per 100 grams), papaya (2,000 milligrams per 100 grams), and strawberry (2,000 milligrams per 100 grams). Other sources of vitamin C include orange, lemon, melon, garlic, cauliflower, grape-fruit, raspberry, tangerine, passion fruit, spinach, and lime. These foods contain about 30 to 50 milligrams per 100 grams of fruits and vegetables. Vitamin C is sold commercially as L-ascorbic acid, calcium ascorbate, sodium ascorbate, and potassium ascorbate.

Carotenoids

The richest sources of carotenoids are sweet potato, carrot, spinach, mango, cantaloupe, apricot, kale, broccoli, parsley, cilantro, pumpkin, winter squash, and fresh thyme. There are two main forms of carotenoids found in nature: alpha-carotene and beta-carotene. Beta-carotene is one of the more than 600 carotenoids found in fruits, vegetables, and plants and represents the more common form of carotenoids. Other carotenes include lutein and lycopene.

Vitamin E

The richest sources of vitamin E include wheat germ oil (215 milligrams per 100 grams), sunflower oil (56 milligrams per 100 grams), olive oil (12 milligrams per 100 grams), almond oil (39 milligrams per 100 grams), hazelnut oil (26 milligrams per 100 grams), walnut oil (20 milligrams per 100 grams), and peanut oil (17 milligrams per 100 grams). The sources for small amounts of vitamin E (0.1 to 2 milligrams per 100 grams) include kiwi fruit, fish, leafy vegetables, and whole grains. In the United States fortified breakfast cereal is an important source of vitamin E. At present, the natural form of vitamin E is primarily extracted from vegetable oil, particularly soybean oil.

Vitamin E exists in eight different forms: four tocopherols (alpha-, beta-, gamma-, and delta-tocopherol), and four tocotrienols (alpha-, beta-, gamma-, and delta-tocotrienol). Alpha-tocopherol has the most biological activity. Vitamin E exists in the natural form, commonly indicated as "d," whereas the synthetic form is referred to as "dl." The stable esterified form of vitamin E is available as alpha-tocopheryl acetate, alpha-tocopheryl succinate, and alpha-tocopheryl nicotinate. The activity of vitamin E is generally expressed in international units (IU). It is determined that 1 IU equals 0.66 milligram of d-alpha-tocopherol, and 1 IU of racemic mixture (dl-form) equals 0.45 milligram of d-tocopherol.

Glutathione

Glutathione is synthesized from three amino acids—L-cysteine, L-glutamic acid, and L-glycine—and is present in all cells of the body; however, its highest concentration is found in the liver. Glutathione exists in the cells in a reduced or oxidized form. In healthy cells more than 90 percent of glutathione is present in the reduced form. The oxidized form of glutathione can be converted to the reduced form by the enzyme glutathione reductase. The reduced form of glutathione acts as an antioxidant.

L-carnitine

L-carnitine was originally found to be a growth factor for mealworms. It is synthesized primarily in the liver and kidneys from the amino acids lysine and methionine. Vitamin C is necessary for its synthesis. It exists as R-L-carnitine, a biologically active form, and as D-carnitine, a biologically inactive form.

Polyphenolic Compounds

Polyphenolic compounds are found in herbs, fruits, vegetables, and plants. They include tannins, lignins, and flavonoids. The most widely studied polyphenolic compounds are flavonoids, which include resveratrol (in grape skin and seed), curcumin (in spices such as turmeric), ginseng extract, cinnamon extract, garlic extract, quercetin, epicatechin, and oligomeric proanthocyanidins. Major sources of flavonoids include all citrus fruit, berries, *Ginkgo biloba,* onion, parsley, tea, red wine, and dark chocolate. More than five thousand naturally occurring flavonoids have been characterized from various plants.

ABSORPTION OF ANTIOXIDANTS

Antioxidants are absorbed from the intestinal tract and then distributed to various organs of the body. The highest levels of vitamins A, C, and E are present in the liver, and the lowest levels of these antioxidants are in the brain. Regarding coenzyme Q10, the heart and the liver have the highest levels of it. Only about 10 percent of ingested water-soluble and fat-soluble antioxidants are absorbed from the intestinal tract. It has been argued by some that 90 percent of antioxidants are therefore wasted, but this argument has no scientific merit.

During the process of digestion, many toxic substances including mutagens (agents that can alter genetic activity) and carcinogens (agents that can cause cancer) are formed. What's interesting to note is that the consumption of organic food makes little difference in the amount of toxins formed during the digestive process. Organic food may, however, be devoid of pesticides, although these pesticides represent only about 1 percent of naturally occurring toxins. Pesticides are not metabolized and are difficult to remove from the body.

The formation of toxins is more prevalent in meat eaters than in vegetarians. A portion of the toxins is absorbed from the gut and could increase the risk of chronic disease developing over a long period of time. The presence of excessive amounts of antioxidants markedly reduced the levels of toxins formed during digestion and thereby reduced the risk of chronic disease development. Thus it is clear that unabsorbed antioxidants perform a very useful function in reducing the levels of mutagens and carcinogens formed during the digestion of food.

SOLUBILITY OF ANTIOXIDANTS AND POLYPHENOLIC COMPOUNDS

The lipid-soluble antioxidants include vitamin A, vitamin E, carotenoids, coenzyme Q10, and L-carnitine. Water-soluble antioxidants include vitamin C, glutathione, and alpha-lipoic acid. Polyphenolic compounds are generally fat-soluble. Fat-soluble vitamins and polyphenolic compounds should be taken with meals so that they are more readily absorbed.

AVAILABILITY OF ANTIOXIDANTS

Vitamin A

Vitamin A is commercially sold as retinyl palmitate, retinyl acetate, and retinoic acid and its analogues. Retinyl acetate or retinyl palmitate is converted to retinol in the intestine before absorption. Retinol is converted to retinoic acid in the cells. Retinoic acid performs all of the functions of vitamin A except for maintaining good vision. Retinol is stored in the liver as retinyl palmitate. Vitamin A exists as a protein-bound molecule. The level of retinol can be determined in the plasma.

Vitamin C

Vitamin C is commercially sold as ascorbic acid, sodium ascorbate, magnesium ascorbate, calcium ascorbate, and timed-release capsules containing ascorbic acid and vitamin C-ester. It is present in all cells. Ascorbic acid is converted to dehydroascorbic acid, which can be reduced to form vitamin C. It's interesting to note that dehydroascorbic acid can cross the blood-brain barrier, but vitamin C cannot. All mammals make vitamin C except guinea pigs. An adult goat makes about thirteen grams of vitamin C every day. The plasma level of vitamin C may not reflect the tissue level of vitamin C, but in humans it's difficult to obtain tissues to determine vitamin C levels. Vitamin C can recycle oxidized vitamin E to the reduced form, which acts as an antioxidant.

Carotenoids

Beta-carotene is one of more than six hundred carotenoids found in fruits, vegetables, and plants. It is commercially available in natural or synthetic forms. The natural form of beta-carotene is more effective than the synthetic form. Preparations of natural carotenoids contain primarily beta-carotene; however, the other type of carotenoid is also present. A portion of ingested beta-carotene is converted to retinol (vitamin A) in the intestinal tract before absorption, and the remainder is distributed in the blood and tissues of the body. One molecule of beta-carotene forms two molecules of vitamin A. In humans the conversion of beta-carotene to vitamin A doesn't occur if the body has sufficient amounts of vitamin A. Beta-carotene is primarily stored in the eyes and fatty tissues. Other carotenoids such as lycopene accumulate in the prostate more than in any other organ, whereas lutein accumulates in the eyes more than in any other organ.

Coenzyme Q10

About 95 percent of energy is generated from the use of coenzyme Q10 by the mitochondria. Therefore, organs such as the heart and liver that require high energy have the highest concentrations of coenzyme Q10. Other organelles inside the cells that contain coenzyme Q10 include endoplasmic reticulum, peroxisomes, lysosomes, and Golgi apparatus.

Vitamin E

Among vitamin E isomers, alpha-tocopherol is biologically more active than others. In recent years the research on tocotrienols has revealed some important biological functions. Vitamin E is commercially sold as d- or dl-tocopherol, alpha-tocopheryl acetate (vitamin E acetate), or alpha-tocopheryl succinate (vitamin E succinate). The esterified forms of vitamin E (vitamin E acetate and vitamin E succinate) are more stable than alpha-tocopherol. Vitamin E acetate has been widely used in basic research and clinical studies.

It's been presumed that vitamin E acetate and vitamin E succinate are converted to alpha-tocopherol in the intestinal tract before absorption. This assumption may be true for vitamin E succinate. If the body's stores of alpha-tocopherol are saturated, vitamin E succinate can be absorbed. Vitamin E succinate enters the cells more easily than alpha-tocopherol because of its greater solubility. As well, vitamin E succinate has some unique functions that cannot be produced by alpha-tocopherol.

Vitamin E succinate is now considered the most effective form of vitamin E, but it cannot act as an antioxidant until it is converted to alpha-tocopherol. Alpha-tocopherol is located primarily in the membranous structures of the cells. The level of vitamin E can be determined in the plasma.

Glutathione and Alpha-Lipoic Acid

Glutathione is the most important antioxidant within the cells, and it is present in all cells. Although it's sold commercially for oral consumption, it's totally destroyed in the intestine. Therefore, oral administration of glutathione doesn't increase the cellular level of glutathione; however, n-acetylcysteine (NAC) does. In the body n-acetyl is removed from NAC by the enzyme esterase, and then cysteine is used to synthesize glutathione.

Alpha-lipoic acid also increases the cellular levels of glutathione by a mechanism that differs from the mechanism of NAC.

L-carnitine

L-carnitine is made in the body, but we can also obtain it from the diet. The highest concentration of L-carnitine is found in red meat (95 milligrams per 3.0 ounces of meat). In contrast, chicken breast has only 3.9 milligrams per 3.5 ounces. L-carnitine is present in all of the cells of our body.

Melatonin

Melatonin is a naturally occurring hormone produced primarily by the pineal gland in the brain. It is also produced by the retina, the lens, and the gastrointestinal tract. Melatonin is synthesized from the amino acid tryptophan. It is also present in various plants such as rice. It is readily absorbed from the intestinal tract; however, 50 percent of it is removed from the plasma in thirty-five to fifty minutes. It has several biological functions including antioxidant and anti-inflammatory activities. Melatonin is necessary for the proper regulation of sleep cycles.

Nicotinamide (Vitamin B₃) and Reduced Nicotinamide Adenine Dinucleotide Dehydrogenase (NADH)

Treatment with nicotinamide, a precursor of nicotinamide adenine dinucleotide (NAD+), reduced oxidative stress-induced mitochondrial dysfunction and increased the survival of neurons in culture. Nicotinamide also attenuated glutamate-induced toxicity. Histone deacetylase inhibitors increase histone acetylation and enhance memory and neuronal plasticity. Nicotinamide (vitamin B₃), an inhibitor of histone deacetylase activity, restored memory deficits in Alzheimer's transgenic mice. Thus, the addition of nicotinamide to a preparation of micronutrients may be necessary to reduce the risk of developing memory loss and to increase the survival of neurons in neurodegenerative diseases.

Nicotinamide adenine dinucleotide (NAD+) and NADH (the reduced form of NAD) are present in all of the cells of our body. NAD+ is an oxidizing agent; therefore, it can act as a prooxidant, whereas NADH can act as an antioxidant. NAD+ accepts electrons from other molecules and is reduced to form NADH. NADH can recycle oxidized vitamin E to the reduced form, which can act as an antioxidant. NADH is essential for mitochondria to generate energy.

Polyphenolic Compounds

Flavonoids (polyphenolic compounds) are poorly absorbed by the intestinal tract in humans. All of them possess varying degrees of antioxidants and anti-inflammatory activities.

HOW TO STORE ANTIOXIDANTS

Vitamin A

Crystal forms of retinol, retinoic acid, retinyl acetate, and retinal palmitate can be stored at 4°C for several months. A solution of retinoic acid is stable at 4°C, stored away from light, for several weeks.

Vitamin C

Vitamin C should not be stored in solution form, because it is easily destroyed within a few days. The crystal or tablet forms of vitamin C can be kept at room temperature, away from light, for a few years.

Carotenoids

Most commercially sold carotenoids in solid form can be stored at room temperature, away from light, for a few years. Beta-carotene in solution, however, degrades within a few days, even when stored in a colder environment away from light.

Coenzyme Q10 and NADH

These antioxidants in solid forms are stable when stored at room temperature, away from light, for few years. The solutions of these antioxidants are stable when stored at 4°C, away from light, for several months.

Vitamin E

Alpha-tocopherol is relatively unstable at room temperature in comparison to alpha-tocopheryl acetate and alpha-tocopheryl succinate. Alpha tocopherol can be stored at 4°C for several weeks, but alpha-tocopheryl acetate and alpha-tocopheryl succinate can be stored at room temperature for a few years. A solution of alpha-tocopheryl succinate is stable for several months at 4°C if kept away from the light.

Glutathione, N-acetylcysteine, and Alpha-Lipoic Acid

Solid forms of glutathione, n-acetylcysteine, and alpha-lipoic acid are stable at room temperature, away from light, for a few years. The solutions of these antioxidants are stable when stored at 4°C, away from light, for several months.

Melatonin

The powdered form of melatonin is stable at 4°C for a year or more.

Polyphenolic Compounds

Polyphenolic compounds are very stable at room temperature, away from light, for a few years.

CAN ANTIOXIDANTS BE DESTROYED DURING COOKING?

Vitamin A

Routine cooking does not destroy vitamin A, but slow heating for a long period of time may reduce its potency. Canning and prolonged cold storage may also diminish its activity. The vitamin A content of fortified milk powder declines substantially after two years.

Carotenoids

Most carotenes, especially lutein and lycopene, are not destroyed during cooking. In fact, their bioavailability improves when they're derived from a cooked or extracted preparation, for example, lycopene from tomato sauce.

Coenzyme Q10 and NADH

Coenzyme Q10 and NADH can be partially degraded during cooking.

Vitamin E

Food processing, frying, and freezing destroy vitamin E. The vitamin E content of fortified milk powder is unaffected over a two-year period.

Glutathione, N-acetylcysteine, and Alpha-Lipoic Acid

Glutathione, n-acetylcysteine, and alpha-lipoic acid can be partially destroyed during cooking.

Polyphenolic Compounds

Polylphenolic compounds are not destroyed during cooking.

TOXICITY OF MICRONUTRIENTS

Some micronutrients may produce harmful effects but only when consumed at relatively high doses over a long period of time. For example, vitamin A at doses of 10,000 IU or more per day can cause birth defects in pregnant women, and beta-carotene at doses of 50 milligrams or more can produce bronzing of the skin that is reversible on discontinuation. Vitamin C as ascorbic acid at high doses (10 grams or more per day) can cause diarrhea in some individuals. Vitamin E at high doses (2,000 IU or more per day) can induce clotting defects after long-term consumption. Vitamin B$_6$ at high doses (50 milligrams or more per day) may produce peripheral neuropathy, and selenium at doses 400 micrograms or more per day can cause skin and liver toxicity after long-term consumption. Coenzyme Q10 has no known toxicity, and recommended daily doses are 30 to 400 milligrams. N-acetylcysteine (NAC) doses of 250 to 1,500 milligrams and alpha-lipoic acid doses of 600 milligrams are used in humans without toxicity.

CURRENT CONTROVERSIES ABOUT ANTIOXIDANTS IN THE PREVENTION OF CHRONIC DISEASE

Despite the fact that antioxidants are so essential for our growth and survival, they remain the most misunderstood and misused molecules by the public and by most health care professionals. The reasons for this include inaccurate claims by many in the nutrition industry, inconsistent human data (stemming from the epidemiologic studies), and the results of poorly designed clinical studies in which one or sometimes two or more dietary antioxidants were administered to populations at high risk for developing chronic disease.

We consume some antioxidants such as vitamin A, carotenoids, vitamin C, and vitamin E from the diet. Other antioxidants, such as glutathione, alpha-lipoic acid, coenzyme Q10, and L-carnitine we make ourselves. Despite basic science evidence for the importance of multiple antioxidants in disease prevention, and improvement in the management of chronic diseases, when these antioxidants are used in combination with standard therapy, medical establishments are not convinced of their efficacy. This is not the first time the medical establishment has resisted the application of novel agents in the treatment of disease. As a matter of fact, the history of the discovery of vitamins A and C illustrates that the cure for night blindness and scurvy was delayed for centuries because of resistance by the medical establishment.

MISUSE OF ANTIOXIDANTS IN CLINICAL STUDIES FOR THE PREVENTION OF CHRONIC DISEASE

Humans need dietary antioxidants (vitamins A, C, E, and carotenoids as well as the mineral selenium) in addition to endogenous antioxidants made by the body. These endogenous antioxidants include antioxidant enzymes, glutathione, coenzyme Q10, alpha-lipoic acid, L-carnitine, reduced nicotinamide adenine dinucleotide (NADH), B vitamins, and certain minerals necessary for growth and survival. The distribution of these antioxidants markedly varies from one organ to another, even within the same cell. Their subcellular distribution differs markedly from one cellular compartment to another within the same cell.

The human body generates different types of inorganic and organic free radicals derived from oxygen and nitrogen in response to the utilization of oxygen. The exposure to various environmental stressors, such as ozone, dust particles, smoke, toxic fumes, toxic chemicals, and ionizing radiation (X-rays or gamma rays) also produces excessive amounts of free radicals. Free radical–induced damage is called oxidative damage. It also occurs during the normal aging process and during the initiation and progression of certain neurodegenerative diseases.

The elevation of dietary and endogenous antioxidant chemicals as well as antioxidant enzymes is needed to reduce oxidative stress and inflammation optimally. The affinities of antioxidants to specific types of free radicals differ, and their efficacy in reducing oxidative damage may also differ. Some antioxidants also reduce the levels of chronic inflammation and reduce glutamate release and its consequent toxicity. Increased oxidative damage, chronic inflammation, and glutamate release are associated with acute and chronic neurodegenerative disease.

These observations make it clear that supplementation with one or two dietary or endogenous antioxidants may not be useful in reducing the progression of damage in patients with acute or chronic neurodegenerative disease. I propose that supplementation with a preparation of micronutrients containing dietary and endogenous antioxidants, B vitamins, vitamin D_3, selenium, and certain phenolic compounds (curcumin, resveratrol, and omega-3-fatty acids) may be essential for reducing the risk of developing as well as of slowing the progression of chronic neurodegenerative disease. Unfortunately nearly all previous clinical studies have utilized just one or two dietary antioxidants in populations at a high risk of developing certain chronic diseases, yielding inconsistent results.

In addition to the above considerations, selection of the type of antioxidants is equally important for any human clinical studies. For example, it has been reported that natural beta-carotene prevented X-ray-induced transformation of normal mouse fibroblasts in culture, whereas synthetic beta-carotene did not. An animal study showed that various organs accumulated the natural form of vitamin E (d-alpha-tocopherol) more than the synthetic form (dl-alpha-tocopherol). Furthermore, it has been reported that vitamin E in the form of d-alpha-tocopheryl succinate is more effective than other forms of vitamin E. The human antioxidant studies that have been published have not taken into consideration these important issues in the design of their experiments; therefore, the results regarding the efficacy of antioxidants have been contradictory.

The doses of antioxidants are very important in order to produce optimal health benefits and disease prevention. Low doses (in the neighborhood of the RDA values) may be useful in reducing some oxidative damage and preventing deficiency; however, they may not be sufficient in reducing inflammation or optimizing immune function. The differences in changes in the expression of gene profiles between low and high doses of an antioxidant are very marked. In commercially sold multivitamin preparations the doses of antioxidants and other micronutrients vary markedly. The selection of appropriate doses of various micronutrients, including dietary and endogenous antioxidants that are safe and standardized, is essential for good health and disease prevention.

The dose schedule of antioxidant micronutrients is also very critical for achieving the desired health benefits. Most people take micronutrient supplements once a day, which may not produce optimal health benefits. This is due to the fact that a high degree of fluctuation in the levels of antioxidants occurs in the body because of variation in the plasma half-lives of various micronutrients. In addition, the expression of gene profiles of cells differs markedly depending upon the level of antioxidants in the body. A once-a-day dose schedule may compel the cells to adjust their genetic activity all the time due to variations in the levels of antioxidants in the body. Such a large fluctuation in the genetic activity may not be desirable for the optimal function of the cells. It's interesting to note that all previous human studies with antioxidants have utilized the once-a-day schedule in spite of scientific evidence that contraindicates its efficacy.

In all human studies with antioxidants, the selection of the target population and the statistical analysis have been appropriate, but the selection of antioxidants, doses, and dose schedule have been without any scientific rationale. This can be demonstrated by a few widely publicized results on antioxidant studies in humans. In a clinical study the synthetic form of beta-carotene was administered orally once a day to male, heavy-tobacco smokers to reduce the incidence of lung cancer. The results showed that the incidence of lung cancer in beta-carotene-treated smokers increased by about 17 percent. Federal agencies and some nutrition scientists then promoted the idea that supplementation with beta-carotene may be harmful to your health and recommended that consumers not take beta-carotene in any form or in any other multiple vitamin preparation. These erroneous conclusions and recommendations were without any scientific merit for the following reasons.

It had been known before the start of this human study that individual antioxidants such as beta-carotene can be oxidized in a high oxidative environment to become a prooxidant. Heavy-tobacco smokers have a high internal oxidative environment. Therefore, when beta-carotene is administered to smokers it is oxidized and acts as a prooxidant rather than as an antioxidant. One would then expect an increase in the incidence of cancer in tobacco smokers.

Knowing the above facts about beta-carotene and heavy-tobacco smokers, one could have predicted that beta-carotene would increase the risk of lung cancer in smokers. Indeed, the results of the trial confirmed this prediction. In contrast to the adverse effects of beta-carotene in heavy-tobacco smokers, the same dose and type of beta-carotene did not increase the risk of cancer among doctors and nurses who were nonsmokers during a five-year follow-up. Again, this result was also expected, because populations of nonsmokers do not have a high internal oxidative environment.

The synthetic form of vitamin E has produced inconsistent results in patients with a high risk of cardiovascular disease who have an increased internal oxidative environment. Some studies showed beneficial effects, whereas others showed no effect or even adverse effects in some cases. Harmful effects of vitamin E alone on cardiovascular disease can be attributed to the same biological events as those observed with beta-carotene. At this time cardiologists do not recommend vitamin E to their patients. There are no human data (intervention studies) to show that the same dose of vitamin E or beta-carotene, when present in an appropriately prepared multiple micronutrient including dietary and endogenous antioxidants, produces adverse health effects among normal or high-risk populations.

The human studies featuring a single antioxidant have also produced inconsistent results in neurological diseases such as Parkinson's disease and Alzheimer's disease. In both studies high doses of the synthetic form of vitamin E at a dose of 800 IU per day in Parkinson's and 2,000 IU per day in Alzheimer's were used. No beneficial effects of vitamin E were observed in Parkinson's, but some beneficial effects were observed in Alzheimer's disease. These studies were begun without careful consideration of the biochemical factors involved in the diseases' processes or antioxidant status in the patients.

It has been reported that deficiency of the antioxidant glutathione rather than vitamin E is found in both Alzheimer's and Parkinson's patients. In addition, dysfunction of the mitochondria is consistently observed in the autopsied samples of the brains of patients with Parkinson's or Alzheimer's disease. Furthermore, evidence of high oxidative damage and chronic inflammation are also found in these brains. Therefore, the idea of supplementation with antioxidants for the prevention and reduction in the rate of progression of disease is a very good one.

Supplementation with a multiple micronutrient preparation that contains appropriate doses of dietary and endogenous antioxidants—including glutathione-elevating agents, as well as antioxidants that improve the ability of mitochondria to generate energy—would have provided better health outcomes than those obtained by vitamin E alone.

It is very unfortunate that the harmful results obtained with the use of primarily one antioxidant in high-risk populations are often extrapolated to all multiple antioxidant preparations and to all populations. This erroneous extrapolation of data regarding the harmful effects of beta-carotene or vitamin E alone is further propagated by the publication of meta-analysis of published data on the same vitamins with the same conclusion. (A meta-analysis publication is often misinterpreted as an original study.) In my opinion a meta-analysis should critically examine an experiment's design instead of just summarizing the results of previous studies. These kinds of experiments and extrapolations have created a wide disconnect between the public and most health care professionals—especially physicians—regarding the health benefits of micronutrients.

To avoid these problems the subsequent chapters in this book discuss the scientific basis for using multiple micronutrients, including dietary and endogenous antioxidants, in healthy aging and in reducing the risk of Parkinson's disease and Huntington's disease. In addition, the role of these micronutrients in improving the efficacy of standard therapy for these neurodegenerative diseases is also discussed.

CONCLUDING REMARKS

Early in the mists of time, when life on the planet consisted primarily of small, anaerobic organisms, oxygen as we know it today did not yet exist. However, these organisms eventually acquired the ability to break down water into its constituent parts of hydrogen and oxygen. Because the newly generated oxygen was toxic to these organisms they had to adapt to it in order to survive. They did this by developing defensive systems that would protect them from oxidative damage. As these organisms evolved into humans, defensive antioxidant shields evolved with them.

When the body processes oxygen, free radicals are created. Infection and metabolism are two additional processes that generate free radicals in the body. As well, certain trace minerals (iron, copper, and manganese), in combination with molecules like vitamin C and uric acid can also form free radicals. These free radicals may overwhelm the body's antioxidant system, thus underscoring the need to ensure the presence of large amounts of antioxidants in the body at all times.

There are many different types of antioxidants: those that are made in the body and those that are derived from outside sources via either diet or dietary supplement. In terms of dietary antioxidants and guidance regarding their consumption, it's useful to refer to the

Daily Recommended Intake, which is an index established for each micronutrient. The DRI is found in the appendix of this book. (The DRI replaces the former index known as the Recommended Dietary Allowances.) However, and it must be noted, that although these recommended doses allow for normal growth and development, they're not optimal for reducing increased oxidative stress and inflammation.

In the next chapter we will take a look at the history, incidence, cost, and causes of Parkinson's disease in an effort to further understand this debilitating disease as we seek to provide prevention and treatment strategies to combat it.

4 Parkinson's Disease
History, Incidence, Cost, and Causes

Parkinson's disease is associated with involuntary tremor of the limbs and trunk as well as with non-motor deficits and neurological symptoms, including an impaired sense of smell, memory loss, and psychiatric symptoms. Parkinson's disease is the second most common form of neurodegenerative disease (Alzheimer's is the first). It is considered to be a slow, progressive, chronic neurodegenerative disease characterized by the loss of dopamine (DA) neurons from the brain. Indeed, pathologists have repeatedly reported that there is a loss of dopamine-producing nerve cells (DA neurons) from the substantia nigra (SN) region of the brain of Parkinson's patients.

Parkinson's disease is also characterized by the presence of Lewy bodies in the cytoplasm of the neuron and its neurites. Lewy bodies are considered consequences of neuronal damage. In addition to the substantia nigra region of the brain, other areas of the brain such as the locus coeruleus, the reticular nuclei of the brain stem, the dorsal motor nucleus of the vagus, and the amygdala and the CA2 neurons of the hippocampus are affected. Lewy bodies are also found in these locations of the brain.

Lewy bodies containing predominantly neurofilaments, alpha-synuclein, and another protein, FOXO3 (a transcriptional activator that can trigger neuronal death upon oxidative stress), were found in

58

the autopsied brain samples of Parkinson's victims as well as in Lewy body dementia (Su et al. 2009).

Lewy bodies can be transferred from one neuron to another by endocytosis (a process of engulfing the materials inside the cells). This was demonstrated by the fact that Lewy bodies were present in neurons grafted in patients with Parkinson's disease and in a transgenic animal model of Parkinson's (Desplats et al. 2009).

It is estimated that in normal individuals about 3 to 5 percent of DA neurons are lost every decade; however, in Parkinson's patients the rate of loss is greater than that found in normal individuals (Mandel et al. 2003). An examination of the autopsied samples of Parkinson's brains revealed that about 70 to 75 percent of DA neurons have been lost by the time the disease becomes detectable. This suggests that DA neurons possess a high degree of functional plasticity. This property of the brain makes it possible for fewer DA neurons to maintain normal motor function. This study also suggests that an early intervention to reduce biochemical defects responsible for the death of DA neurons may decrease the rate of loss of DA neurons and thereby may prevent the onset of Parkinson's disease.

Currently there is no known cure for Parkinson's disease, but certain drugs, namely levodopa and carbidopa, have proved effective in relieving its symptoms in a large majority of persons afflicted. In combination these drugs act to generate dopamine in the diseased brain, which is in short supply due to the nature of the disease. This drug protocol of levodopa and carbidopa is typically used for a period lasting no longer than five years due to the toxic effects of some after the five-year window has expired. Surgery is another viable option. (A longer discussion of the medical and surgical options available to treat Parkinson's follows in later chapters of this book.)

Research on Parkinson's disease has identified some environmental-, dietary-, and lifestyle-related factors that influence its incidence. In order to develop rational strategies for the prevention and improved management of Parkinson's it's essential to identify some major biochemical defects that participate in its development and progression. These defects include increased oxidative stress, mitochondrial dysfunction, chronic inflammation, and proteasome inhibition. The major genetic defects include overexpression of alpha-synuclein, or mutation in alpha-synuclein, and mutations in DJ-1, PARKIN, and PINK1 genes.

This chapter briefly describes the history, incidence and prevalence, cost, and pathology (progressive damage to the nerve cells) of the brain, as well as the symptoms and causes of Parkinson's disease. Herein we also propose that increased oxidative stress is one of the earliest biochemical defects that initiate degeneration in DA neurons. Other biochemical defects occur subsequent to increased oxidative stress. Genetic defects associated with individuals with a family history of Parkinson's are detailed as well.

HISTORY OF PARKINSON'S DISEASE

The symptoms of Parkinson's disease have been known for thousands of years, initially surfacing in the ancient Indian medical practice of ayurveda, which has been in existence since 5000 BCE. A tropical legume by the name of *Mucuna pruriens,* which was referred to as Atmagupta in the ancient ayurvedic texts, was used to treat its symptoms. This legume is a natural source of the therapeutic quantities of L-dopa (dopamine) that are clinically used today in the treatment of Parkinson's disease.

An Egyptian papyrus from the twelfth century BCE articulates that the kings of Egypt drooled in older age, and the Bible contains a number of references to various individuals who displayed signs of tremor. Symptoms of Parkinson's disease were also mentioned in a Chinese medical text titled *Neijing* more than twenty-five hundred years ago. In 175 CE a Greek physician by the name of Galen described the disease as "shaking palsy." In 1817, Dr. James Parkinson of England published a detailed account of shaking palsy.

Approximately sixty years later French physician Dr. Jean Martin Charcot recognized the importance of Dr. Parkinson's research and named the disease after him.

PREVALENCE, INCIDENCE, AND COST OF PARKINSON'S DISEASE

Prevalence and Incidence

The term *prevalence* in a medical context is a measurement of how many cases of a disease exist in the population in a given time frame, whereas *incidence* refers to the number of cases of a disease that *develop* every year. In the United States approximately 1 million people suffer from Parkinson's disease, and approximately 60,000 new cases are diagnosed annually (Parkinson's Disease Foundation, 2013). Approximately 3 million to 4 million people remain undiagnosed.

The average age that individuals develop Parkinson's is sixty, and approximately 4 percent of people with the disease are diagnosed before the age of fifty. The incidence of Parkinson's increases with age. Men are 1.5 times more likely to develop Parkinson's than are women. The age-sex-adjusted annual incidence rates in ethnic groups were highest among Hispanics, followed by non-Hispanic whites, Asians, and blacks (Van Den Eeden et al. 2003). The data are summarized below.

TABLE 4.1. INCIDENCE OF PARKINSON'S DISEASE IN THE UNITED STATES

Ethnic Group	Incidence (cases/100,000 people)
Non-Hispanic White	13.6
Hispanic	16.6
Asian	11.3
Black	10.2

Worldwide approximately 6.3 million people have Parkinson's disease. The World Health Organization (WHO) estimates that the prevalence of Parkinson's is roughly 160 cases per 100,000 individuals. The annual incidence of this disease is about 16 to 19 cases per 100,000 (International Group of Researchers and Development for Complementary Medicine, 2013).

Cost

In the United States, the direct and indirect cost of Parkinson's disease is estimated to be approximately $25 billion per year. The average per person medical cost is roughly $2,500 per year, and the cost of therapeutic surgery may be as high as $100,000 per patient (Parkinson's Disease Foundation, 2013).

SYMPTOMS OF PARKINSON'S DISEASE

The major symptoms of Parkinson's include tremor, muscle rigidity, postural problems, gait disorders, speaking difficulties, cognitive dysfunction, and immobility—leading to total disability and death. The non-motor symptoms include sleep disorders due to a dysfunctional circadian system. This could be due to a defect in the signaling output from the suprachiasmatic nuclei caused by increased oxidative stress and mitochondrial dysfunction (Willison et al. 2013).

CAUSES OF PARKINSON'S DISEASE

Identifying agents that can increase or decrease the risk of developing Parkinson's—including external factors related to diet and lifestyle as well as internal biochemical defects—is important in developing rational strategies for its prevention and improved management.

EXTERNAL FACTORS THAT INFLUENCE
THE DEVELOPMENT OF PARKINSON'S DISEASE

Age

Advanced age (over the age of sixty) is a risk factor for idiopathic Parkinson's.

Exposure to Toxic Substances

Exposure to an excess of manganese (Mn) produces cognitive dysfunction (memory loss), motor deficits (involuntary tremors), and psychiatric problems. Welders exposed to high levels of manganese from welding fumes exhibited abnormal functioning of DA neurons. In addition, smelter workers who were exposed to manganese showed defects in the function of the thalamus and frontal cortex regions of the brain (Racette et al. 2012).

An epidemiologic (survey-type) study on manganese miners showed an increased incidence of Parkinson's-like syndromes (Mena et al. 1969). This may be due to the fact that the brains of manganese miners accumulate increased levels of free manganese, which can enhance the production of free radicals. This then gradually causes damage to DA neurons.

A review of 104 research studies with 3,087 references revealed that the risk of Parkinson's increased among individuals who were exposed to pesticides, herbicides, or certain solvents (Pezzoli and Cereda 2013). Exposure to fungicides did not increase the risk (van der Mark et al. 2012).

Some organic solvents also can increase the risk of developing Parkinson's. For example, trichloroethylene (TCE) is the most common organic contaminant in groundwater, whereas perchloroethylene (PERC) and carbon tetrachloride (CCl) are ubiquitous in the environment. Among these solvents TCE was the most effective in increasing the risk of Parkinson's (Goldman et al. 2012).

Paraquat, one of the herbicides, as well as neonatal iron exposure also increased the risk; however, a combination of paraquat and iron increased damage to DA neurons via increased oxidative stress in a synergistic manner (Peng et al. 2009).

Recreational Drug Use

In 1980 an increased incidence of Parkinson's-like syndrome was seen among users of the designer drug meperidene, which contains 1-methyl-4-phenyl 1,2,3,6 tetrahydropyridine (MPTP), a neurotoxic by-product formed during the synthesis of this drug (Ballard, Tetrud, and Langston 1985). At least one of the mechanisms of action of MPTP-induced degeneration of DA neurons is mediated by free radicals.

Cigarettes: An epidemiologic (survey-type) study suggested that cigarette smoking may reduce the risk of developing Parkinson's disease. To clarify the role of smoking, a clinical study was performed on 113 pairs of twins in which at least one twin (of a pair) had Parkinson's. The results showed that cigarette smoking reduced the risk. The reduction in the incidence of Parkinson's was most pronounced in genetically identical twins (Tanner et al. 2002).

Ibuprofen: An epidemiologic study showed that ibuprofen users, but not aspirin (acetylsalicylic acid) users, had a reduced risk of Parkinson's (Samii et al. 2009).

Caffeine: An epidemiologic study suggested that increased consumption of caffeine decreased the risk of Parkinson's (Hancock et al. 2007).

A combination of cigarette smoking, coffee drinking, and the ingestion of nonsteroidal anti-inflammatory drugs (NSAIDs) was associated with an 87 percent reduction in the incidence of Parkinson's disease (Powers et al. 2008). (I would not recommend cigarette smoking to reduce the risk of Parkinson's, however, because of its overall adverse health effects.)

Nuts and oils: Although no particular dietary risk factors for Parkinson's disease were identified, the consumption of nuts and salad oil (pressed from seeds) appeared to be of protective value against its development (Golbe, Farrell, and Davis 1988).

Vitamin E: Vitamin E consumption was found to be lower among patients with Parkinson's than among normal healthy individuals (control) (de Rijk et al. 1997). (The role of dietary and endogenous antioxidants as they pertain to Parkinson's are discussed in chapter 5.)

INTERNAL BIOCHEMICAL DEFECTS THAT INCREASE THE RISK OF PARKINSON'S DISEASE

Internal biochemical defects in the body that can increase the risk of the development and progression of Parkinson's include increased oxidative stress, mitochondrial dysfunction, chronic inflammation, proteasome inhibition, and defects in certain genes. The evidence for the role of these internal biochemical and genetic defects is discussed below.

EVIDENCE FOR INCREASED OXIDATIVE STRESS IN PARKINSON'S DISEASE

Studies of Autopsied Human Brain Tissue

Several studies have demonstrated the presence of high levels of oxidative stress in the autopsied brain samples of Parkinson's patients. Of all the organs of the body, the normal brain has the highest concentration of unsaturated fatty acids, and these fatty acids are easily damaged by free radicals. Indeed, high levels of oxidative damage have been observed in the autopsied samples of the substantia nigra of diseased brains (Dexter et al. 1994; Ebadi, Srinivasan, and Baxi 1996).

Autopsied samples of the substantia nigra of Parkinson's brains contained reduced levels of antioxidant enzymes and antioxidants (Kish, Morito, and Hornykiewicz 1985; Sofic et al. 2006). The levels of antioxidant glutathione levels were reduced in the substantia nigra of the autopsied brain samples of Parkinson's patients, indicating the presence of high oxidative stress (Fitzmaurice et al. 2003). Increased oxidative stress can impair mitochondrial function.

The levels of oxidative damage as measured by isofurans (products of peroxidation) were elevated in the autopsied samples of the substantia nigra of Parkinson's patients (Fessel et al. 2003).

Heme oxygenase-1 (HO-1) is a cellular stress protein expressed in the brain and other tissues; it becomes elevated in response to increased oxidative stress. The expression of HO-1 was increased in the autopsied samples of the substantia nigra of diseased brains (Schipper, Liberman, and Stopa 1998), suggesting the presence of increased oxidative stress in the brains of Parkinson's patients.

Several studies have confirmed that Parkinson's disease is associated with a significant increase in free iron in the degenerating substantia nigra (Andersen 2004).

The effects of free iron on the degeneration of DA neurons are via increased oxidative stress. The mechanisms of accumulation of iron in the substantia nigra are unknown. The fact that the levels of divalent metal transporter-1 (DMT1) protein are elevated in the substantia nigra of Parkinson's brains (Salazar et al. 2008) suggests that this protein may be responsible for delivering excessive amounts of free iron to the brain.

Glutamate is a major excitatory neurotransmitter in the brain and is toxic to the nerve cells (neurotoxic) when released in excessive amounts. With the loss of DA neurons, the glutamatergic projections from the subthalamic nucleus to the basal ganglia output nuclei become overactive (Blandini, Porter, and Greenamyre 1996) and can release excessive amounts of glutamate.

It has been reported that melanin granules accumulate in the neurons of the substantia nigra of Parkinson's patients. The melanin granules are formed from the auto-oxidation of DA in the substantia nigra of the Parkinson's brain and contain significant amounts of iron (Enochs et al. 1994). The melanin granules can cause degeneration of DA neurons by generating excessive amounts of hydrogen peroxide (H_2O_2) when they are intact or by releasing free iron if they are disintegrated. In addition, dying DA neurons can release melanin granules that can initiate chronic inflammatory responses by activating microglia cells in the brain.

Uric acid in the blood exhibits antioxidant activity. Serum uric acid levels were lower in Parkinson's patients than in healthy individuals in a Chinese population (control), suggesting the presence of increased oxidative stress in the brain. The levels of uric acid correlated with the progression of the disease (Zhang et al. 2012). A similar association between the uric acid levels and disease progression was found in both men and women.

Studies of Human Peripheral Tissue

The levels of markers of oxidative damage and vitamin E were measured in 211 patients with Parkinson's disease and 135 healthy controls. The results showed that the levels of 8-hydroxyguanosine in the leukocytes and malondialdehyde (MDA) in the plasma were elevated, whereas erythrocyte glutathione peroxidase and plasma vitamin E levels were reduced in Parkinson's patients compared to those found in healthy individuals (control) (Sanyal et al. 2009).

The urine levels of 8-hydroxy-2'deoxyguanosine (8-OHdG) and the ratio of OHdG/2-dG were higher in patients with Parkinson's disease than in healthy control subjects; however, only the plasma levels of OHdG/2-dG increased in patients with Parkinson's compared to that of healthy control subjects (Bolner et al. 2011)

It has been reported that the levels of NADH (the reduced form of nicotinamide adenine dehydrogenase) in the platelets of Parkinson's patients were lower compared to healthy age-sex-matched controls, whereas the activity of succinate dehydrogenase was similar in both groups (Varghese et al. 2009).

Plasma levels of vitamin C and vitamin E were decreased in patients with vascular Parkinson's disease (Paraskevas et al. 2003).

In contrast to the above studies, the serum levels of vitamin A, vitamin C, and vitamin E in Parkinson's patients did not differ from that found in healthy individuals (controls) (Fernandez-Calle et al. 1993; Paraskevas et al. 2003).

These studies suggest that serum or plasma levels of vitamin A, vitamin C, or vitamin E should not be used as a marker of oxidative stress in the brain, because they did not reflect the brain levels of antioxidants. Thus, brain tissue levels of antioxidants rather than the blood levels of antioxidants may play a significant role in the development and progression of both spontaneously occurring (idiopathic) Parkinson's disease and familial Parkinson's.

Studies of the Brain in an Animal Model of Parkinson's Disease

It was demonstrated that the expression of divalent metal transporter-1 (DMT1) protein and the levels of iron increased in a MPTP model of rat Parkinson's. These two biological events were associated with increased oxidative stress and neuronal death (Salazar et al. 2008).

The mutation in the DMT1 gene protected rats against toxicity produced by MPTP or 6-hydroxydopamine. It has been reported that treatment with manganese enhanced DA-induced cell death in DA neurons in culture (Prabhakaran et al. 2008).

The effect of manganese is mediated by induction of NF-kappaB and activation of nitric oxide synthase that generates increased amounts of free radicals. Excessive production of NO by treatment with MPTP plays a significant role in the degeneration of DA neurons, because nitric oxide can be oxidized to form peroxynitrite, a form of nitrogen-derived free radical that is highly neurotoxic. Therefore, the involvement of NO in the pathophysiology (progressive damage in the brain) of Parkinson's disease has been proposed (Ebadi and Sharma 2003).

The NADH oxidases (NOXs) are one of the sources of reactive oxygen species (ROS). Therefore, the levels of these enzymes should be elevated in Parkinson's disease. Indeed, the levels of NOX-1 in rat dopamine neurons (N27 cell line) were increased after treatment with 6-hydroxydopamine. Injection of 6-hydroxydopamine directly into the striatum increased the levels of NOX-1 in the DA neurons of the rat substantia nigra. Elevated levels of NOX-1 were also found in the DA neurons of the substantia nigra in autopsied human brain tissues (Choi et al. 2012).

The studies discussed above in human Parkinson's and animal models of Parkinson's disease suggest that increased oxidative stress is one of the biochemical defects that initiates its development. Therefore, reducing oxidative stress is a rational choice for decreasing the risk of developing Parkinson's.

DEFECTS IN MITOCHONDRIAL FUNCTIONS IN PARKINSON'S DISEASE

The mitochondria are the primary site of free radical production; they are also easily damaged by free radicals. Damaged mitochondria produce more free radicals and release cytochrome c, both of which are toxic to nerve cells. Thus, defects in mitochondrial function play a central role in most neurodegenerative diseases including Parkinson's (Arduino et al. 2009); however, they occur subsequent to increased oxidative stress and participate in the disease's development and progression.

Defects in mitochondrial function can be induced by diverse groups of external and internal agents. External agents include MPTP, insecticides, and pesticides, whereas internal agents include increased oxidative stress and chronic inflammation, mutated or aggregated alpha-synuclein, and mutated PINK1, DJ-1, and PARKIN genes (Dodson and Guo 2007; Gautier, Kitada, and Shen 2008; Lee 2003).

Mitochondrial dysfunctions include the following: (a) an impaired electron transport chain responsible for generating energy, (b) mutations in mitochondrial DNA, (c) impaired calcium-buffering ability, (d) reduced energy production, and (e) an abnormal structure of mitochondria (Banerjee et al. 2009).

The consequences of mitochondrial dysfunction include the following: (a) increased oxidative stress, (b) release of cytochrome c, (c) activation of caspase enzyme, (d) chronic inflammation, (e) release of calcium, (f) increased levels of Bax expression and its translocation to mitochondria, and (g) proteasome inhibition—all of which contribute to the degeneration of DA neurons and eventually to their death (Arduino et al. 2009; Domingues et al. 2008). The importance of mitochondrial dysfunction in the pathogenesis (progressive damage in the brain) of Parkinson's disease is further suggested by the fact that rotenone, an inhibitor of mitochondrial complex-1, induces clinical and biochemical features of human Parkinson's in an animal model. Thus, reducing oxidative stress by antioxidants should protect mitochondria and thereby reduce the risk of its development and progression.

THE ROLE OF GLUTAMATE IN PARKINSON'S DISEASE

In the animal model of Parkinson's, inhibitors of glutamate receptors reduced involuntary tremor (abnormality in motor movements) (Bonsi et al. 2007).

Chronic treatment of mice with MPTP increased glutamate levels in the substantia nigra of the brain. Increased glutamate levels contribute to the death of DA neurons (Meredith et al. 2009).

Antioxidants block the toxic effects of glutamate (Schubert, Kimura, and Maher 1992; Sandhu et al. 2003); therefore, they should be useful in improving some of the symptoms of Parkinson's.

EVIDENCE FOR INCREASED CHRONIC INFLAMMATION IN PARKINSON'S DISEASE: HUMAN STUDIES

Microglia in the brain are considered inflammatory cells. In Parkinson's disease microglia are activated, which produce free radicals, pro-inflammatory cytokines, and other toxic products that participate in the degeneration of DA neurons (McGeer and McGeer 2008).

Alpha-synuclein damaged by free radicals activates microglia, which contributes to the degeneration of DA neurons by releasing pro-inflammatory cytokines and other toxic agents (Reynolds et al. 2008).

Activated microglia also can damage alpha-synuclein by releasing excessive amounts of nitric oxide and superoxide. Abnormal alpha-synuclein (excessive amounts of alpha-synuclein or mutated forms of alpha-synuclein) causes degeneration of DA neurons in a transgenic mouse model of Parkinson's (Gao et al. 2008).

In the autopsied brain samples of Parkinson's brains, the number of activated microglia cells increased in the substantia nigra during the disease's progression. The levels of pro-inflammatory cytokines IL-6 and TNF-alpha increased in both Parkinson's and Lewy body disease (Sawada, Imamura, and Nagatsu 2006).

An examination of the autopsied samples of substantia nigra from Parkinson's patients suggests that primarily neurons containing melanin granules are lost (Wilms et al. 2007).

Indeed, pathologists have consistently observed depigmentation of the substantia nigra in the autopsied samples of diseased brains. Treatment of microglia in culture with human brain melanin granules activated the pro-inflammatory transcription factor NF-kappaB (Wilms et al. 2007) and increased the levels of TNF-alpha, IL-6, and nitric oxide. These results suggest that the presence of melanin granules outside the nerve cells serves as a source of chronic inflammation that aggravates the rate of degeneration of DA neurons.

It has been reported that cyclooxygenase (COX) is the rate-limiting enzyme in the synthesis of prostaglandins (PGs), which are toxic to nerve cells in excessive amounts (Prasad, La Rosa, and Prasad 1998). The levels of COX-2 are increased in the DA neurons of autopsied brain samples of Parkinson's patients. The levels of COX-2 are also increased in chemically induced animal Parkinson's models. The enhanced levels of COX-2 in human neuroblastoma cells facilitated oxidation of DA and proteins, including alpha-synuclein (Chae et al. 2008).

The studies presented above clearly show that products of chronic inflammation play an important role in the degeneration and death of DA neurons in Parkinson's disease. Therefore, reducing chronic inflammation appears to be one of the rational choices for reducing the risk of its development and progression.

MUTATIONS OR OVEREXPRESSION IN CERTAIN GENES INCREASE THE RISK OF PARKINSON'S DISEASE

Mutations in six genes have been identified in familial (individuals with a family history) Parkinson's. Mutations in alpha-synuclein (SNCA), PARKIN, PTEN-induced kinase 1 (PINK1), DJ-1, and leucin-rich repeat kinase 2 (LRRK2) are associated with familial Parkinson's disease (Gandhi, Chen, and Wilson-Delfosse 2009; Giaime et al. 2010; Fitzgerald and Plun-Favreau 2008; Dodson and Guo 2007) and account for about 2 to 3 percent of all cases.

In addition, the levels of ATP13A2 gene, which encodes a lysosomal ATPase, increased in the brains of patients with spontaneously occurring Parkinson's (Klein and Lohmann-Hedrich 2007). Transgenic animal models confirm the role of these mutations in its pathology (progressive damage in the brain) (Li et al. 2009; Giasson and Van Deerlin 2008).

Among familial Parkinson's, mutations in the PARKIN gene account for about 50 percent, PINK1 8 to 15 percent, and DJ-1 about 1 percent of cases (da Costa 2007). The mutation in the LRRK2 gene is involved not only in familial Parkinson's but also in some cases of the spontaneously occurring disease.

Overexpression or Mutation of Alpha-Synuclein Gene

The overexpression of the wild-type (normal) alpha-synuclein gene caused degenerative changes in human DA neurons in culture (Zhou et al. 2002) and in transgenic rat DA neurons (Galvin 2006).

The overexpression of human wild-type alpha-synuclein in DA neurons decreased their viability and increased their sensitivity to oxidative stress and neurotoxins such as H_2O_2, nitric oxide, and prostaglandin E2 (Prasad et al. 2004).

Increased oxidative stress, proteasome inhibition, and endoplasmic reticulum stress enhanced the expression of wild-type alpha-synuclein expression in the fibroblasts obtained from patients with Parkinson's disease compared to those obtained from normal individuals (Hoepken et al. 2008).

Increased oxidative stress also caused aggregation of alpha-synuclein, which is toxic to DA neurons. It has been shown that not only insoluble aggregated alpha-synuclein but also soluble oligomer aggregates of alpha-synuclein are toxic to DA neurons (Kalia et al. 2013).

The mechanisms of action of abnormal alpha-synuclein are not well understood, however, it has been suggested that abnormal alpha-synuclein-induced neurotoxicity (damage to the DA neurons) is related to increased oxidative stress (el-Agnaf and Irvine 2002).

Alpha-synuclein enters both outer and inner mitochondrial membranes (Devi and Anandatheerthavarada 2010), and excessive accumulation of alpha-synuclein damages mitochondrial functions, which in turn participate in the degeneration of DA neurons via free radicals and the release of cytochrome c.

The overexpression of human wild-type alpha-synuclein and mutant alpha-synuclein (A30P and A53T) in human neuroblastoma cells in culture enhanced the aggregation of alpha-synuclein, which is toxic to these cells (Parihar et al. 2009).

Dopamine metabolite, 3, 4-dihydroxyphenylacetaldehyde also causes aggregation of alpha-synuclein (Galvin 2006). The aggregated form of alpha-synuclein plays an important role in the pathogenesis of Parkinson's disease (Junn et al. 2009). Mitochondrial dysfunction can also induce alpha-synuclein oligomerization through increased protein oxidation and microtubule depolymerization (damage to microtubules) (Esteves et al. 2009).

Alpha-synuclein-knockout mice (mice with deleted alpha-synuclein) developed normally, but these mice were resistant to MPTP-induced degeneration of DA neurons. In addition, genetic ablation of alpha-synuclein protected neuronal cells in culture against oxidative stress (Junn et al. 2009). Genetic ablation of alpha-synuclein also increased the resistance of human DA neurons to 1-methy-4-phenylpyridine (MPP+) (Wu et al. 2009).

Conversely, overexpression of wild-type alpha-synuclein and mutant alpha-synuclein (A3OP andA53T) increased the sensitivity of neurons to MPP+, which induced mitochondrial dysfunction. It also increased the sensitivity of neurons to 6-hydroxydopamine, which increased oxidative stress in human neuroblastoma cells in culture (Ma et al. 2010).

Alpha-synuclein can be degraded by proteasome and by autophagic (lysosomal) pathways (Kim and Lee 2008). Because of this, any defects in proteasome activity, lysosomal function, or both, can lead to an accumulation of alpha synuclein in the neurons.

An increase in the cellular concentration of alpha-synuclein can lead to its aggregation. The aggregated form of alpha-synuclein plays a central role in the degeneration of DA neurons (Kim and Lee 2008).

It has been demonstrated that increased levels of alpha-synuclein and a nuclear transcriptional factor 2 (Nrf2) deficiency cooperate in the aggregation of alpha-synuclein and induce chronic inflammation in the brain. This caused the death of the brain's nerve cells in mice (Lastres-Becker et al. 2012).

It has been reported that expression of full-length alpha-synuclein caused activation of microglia and induction of MHCII and neurode-generation in mice, whereas in MHCII-knockout mice (mice lacking the MHCII gene) alpha-synuclein did not activate microglia and prevented degeneration of DA neurons (Harms et al. 2013). This suggested that MCHII is necessary for the toxicity of alpha-synuclein in the nerve cells.

Mutated DJ-1 Gene

DJ-1, originally identified as an oncogene, exhibits diverse biological functions, including protection against oxidative stress. It regulates antioxidant-mediated gene expression (Kahle, Waak, and Gasser 2009).

The levels of wild-type DJ-1 can be increased by antioxidant treat-ment in rats (Nunome et al. 2008). Human DJ-1 binds with copper and mercury and thereby prevents metal-induced toxicity in DA neurons (Bjorkblom et al. 2013). DJ-1 acts as a stress sensor, and its levels increase in response to increased oxidative stress (Ariga et al. 2013). DJ-1 is very sensitive to oxidative stress, and the oxidized form of DJ-1 is considered a biomarker for neurodegenerative diseases, including spontaneously occur-ring Parkinson's (Bandopadhyay et al. 2004). The oxidized form of DJ-1 has been found in the autopsied brain tissues of spontaneously occurring Parkinson's disease as well as familial Parkinson's (Kitamura et al. 2011).

Overexpression of wild-type DJ-1 made nerve cells more resistant to oxidative stress induced by H_2O_2 (Gu et al. 2009), protected neurons against DA- and 6-hydroxydopamine-induced toxicity, and reduced intracellular levels of reactive oxygen species (ROS) (Lev et al. 2009).

Mutations in DJ-1 and PARKIN genes made animals more sensitive to oxidative stress and mitochondrial toxins. These mutated genes are involved in spontaneously occurring Parkinson's. Mutated DJ-1 make DA neurons more vulnerable to oxidative stress–induced apoptosis (cell death) (Xu et al. 2005).

Mutated DJ-1 may also promote the aggregation of alpha-synuclein that impairs mitochondrial function, causing DA neurons to degenerate slowly (Batelli et al. 2008).

Loss of DJ-1 leads to mitochondrial dysfunction and fragmentation in human DA neurons via increased oxidative stress (Thomas et al. 2011). This is supported by the fact that treatment with the anti-oxidant n-acetylcysteine reversed the above effects of DJ-1. DJ-1 also protects mitochondrial damage produced by rotenone, a mitochondrial toxin. Overexpression of PARKIN protected against the loss of DJ-1.

The novel compound comp-23 binds with DJ-1. Treatment with comp-23 prevented oxidative stress–induced neuronal death, but it failed to do so in neurons lacking DJ-1, suggesting that the neuroprotective action of comp-23 requires the presence of DJ-1 (Kitamura et al. 2011). Comp-23 also prevented the death of DA neurons in the substantia nigra and restored movement disorders in 6-hydroxydopamine-injected and rotenone-treated Parkinson's model rats and mice.

The vesicular monoamine tranporter-2 (VMAT-2) transfers dopamine into synaptic vesicles for its release and thereby prevents its damage by free radicals. It has been reported that overexpression of DJ-1 protected DA neurons and the vesicular sequestration of dopamine by enhancing the levels of VMAT-2 (Lev et al. 2013). Thus, DJ-1 acts as a regulator of VMAT-2. It has been reported that the nuclear pool of DJ-1 increased in DA neurons after treatment with 6-hydroxydopamine, whereas its level decreased in the cytoplasm.

Treatment with n-acetylcysteine blocked the 6-hydroxydopamine-induced translocation of DJ-1 from the cytoplasm to the nucleus (Kim et al. 2012). This suggests that increased oxidative stress may be involved in the translocation of DJ-1 from the cytoplasm to the nucleus. 6-hydroxydopamine treatment of DA neurons failed to translocate mutant DJ-1 from the cytoplasm to the nucleus. This suggests that only the normal form of DJ-1 responds to increased oxidative stress and that translocation of DJ-1 from the cytoplasm to the nucleus is necessary for the protection of the nerve cells.

Mutated PTEN-Induced Putative Kinase 1 (PINK1) Gene

PINK1 is a ubiquitous protein expressed throughout the human brain and is primarily located in the mitochondrial membrane and the cytoplasm. One of the functions of wild-type (normal) PINK1 is to protect the mitochondria against a variety of stress-signaling pathways, including increased oxidative stress. Genetic ablation of normal PINK1 causes a loss of mitochondrial function (Gegg et al. 2009).

Impairment of mitochondrial function causes damage to mitochondrial DNA; this has been found in the substantia nigra of Parkinson's brains that have been autopsied. PINK1 is also present in Lewy bodies (Gandhi et al. 2006).

Like mutated alpha-synuclein, mutated PINK1 also impaired mitochondrial function. Mutant PINK1 (W437X) enhanced the levels of mutant synuclein (A53T)-induced mitochondrial dysfunction. This effect was associated with increased intracellular calcium levels (Marongiu et al. 2009).

Mutant PINK1 or PINK1 knockdown (deletion of PINK1) reduced mitochondrial function, inhibited proteasome activity, and increased alpha-synuclein aggregation in neuronal cells in culture (Liu et al. 2009).

Mutated PINK1 increased oxidative damage in the fibroblasts obtained from Parkinson's patients (Hoepken et al. 2008).

Mutated PARKIN Gene

The normal PARKIN gene is considered one of the most important factors in improving mitochondrial dysfunction (Mitsui, Kuroda, and Kaji 2008). Normal PINK1 and PARKIN play a central role in the regulation of mitochondrial structures and functions (fission, fusion, migration, and energy generation); therefore, mutations in these genes can impair mitochondrial structure and function (Bueler 2009). Mitochondrial dysfunction interferes with the generation of energy and produces more free radicals. This initiates degeneration of DA neurons and eventually causes neuronal death.

Nitric oxide and oxidative stress inhibit the PARKIN function that may be involved in the pathogenesis of sporadic Parkinson's. To define the role of the PARKIN gene further, stem cells from normal individuals, and patients with mutated PARKIN genes, were established. The results showed that the loss of the PARKIN gene in human DA neurons increased production of monoamine oxidases and the levels of oxidative stress, reduced DA uptake, and enhanced the spontaneous release of DA. Insertion of a wild-type PARKIN gene into these DA neurons prevented the above changes. These results suggest that the PARKIN gene controls dopamine utilization in human DA neurons by increasing the precision of DA neurotransmission and suppressing DA oxidation (Jiang et al. 2012).

Mutated Lysosomal Gene SMPD1

Parkinson's patients with Ashkenazi Jewish ancestry exhibited a strong association between the mutation of SMPD1 (p.L302P), a lysosomal enzyme gene, and an increased risk. This study suggests that defects in the activities of lysosomal enzymes may participate in the disease's pathogenesis (Gan-Or et al. 2013).

CONCLUDING REMARKS

A loss of dopamine neurons in the brain characterizes individuals with Parkinson's disease, which is a chronic, progressive neurodegenerative disease associated with involuntary tremor of the limbs and trunk as well as with non-motor deficits and various neurological symptoms. An impaired sense of smell, memory loss, and mental disorders are some of the presenting symptoms of the disease. In America, 1 million people currently have Parkinson's disease, and another 60,000 people are diagnosed with it annually; men are 1.5 times more likely to develop the disease than women. The age-sex-adjusted annual incidence rate in ethnic groups is highest among Hispanics. This is followed by non-Hispanic whites, Asians, and blacks. In the United States the direct and indirect costs of Parkinson's disease are approximately $25 billion annually.

As we have seen, environmental-, dietary-, and lifestyle-related factors impact the development of Parkinson's disease. Biochemical defects such as increased oxidative stress, mitochondrial dysfunction, chronic inflammation, glutamate release, and proteasome inhibition also participate in Parkinson's. Genetic defects that contribute to the development and progression of the disease include an overexpression of alpha-synuclein or mutation in alpha-synuclein and mutations in DJ-1, PARKIN, and PINK1 genes. More than 95 percent of Parkinson's disease is considered idiopathic. (This means that it occurs sporadically and/or spontaneously and from an unknown cause.) An overexpression of alpha-synuclein or mutations in alpha-synuclein increase the risk of Parkinson's that occurs spontaneously. Mutations in DJ-1, PARKIN, and PINK1 are primarily associated with a family history (familial Parkinson's). To reduce the risk of developing Parkinson's disease and to arrest its progression, it's necessary to reduce oxidative stress and chronic inflammation in the human body.

We will detail specific ways to do this in the following chapters, beginning with the next chapter wherein we will explore the very important role that vitamins and antioxidants play in reducing the risk of and managing Parkinson's disease.

5 Prevention and Management of Parkinson's Disease with Vitamins and Antioxidants

In the previous chapter we discussed the prevalence of Parkinson's disease in the world, noting that the average age of developing this disease is age sixty. As baby boomers continue to age, the prevalence of this disease is likely to increase significantly. Therefore, novel strategies based on the causes of Parkinson's disease should be developed for its prevention and improved management.

As we have already established, reducing oxidative stress and chronic inflammation may be one of the rational choices for reducing the risk of developing Parkinson's disease. The same strategy in combination with standard therapy may improve its management more than that produced by standard therapy alone. To reduce oxidative stress and chronic inflammation optimally it's essential to elevate the levels of antioxidant enzymes (glutathione peroxidase, catalase, and superoxide dismutase), as well as dietary and endogenous antioxidants, in the body.

At present there is no effective strategy to reduce the incidence of Parkinson's in high-risk populations (individuals with a family history and individuals over the age of sixty-five). Current therapeutic approaches are based on the symptoms rather than the causes of the disease. Drug and surgical treatments are very effective in improving the major symptoms, but the benefits of these treatments are only transient. The drug levodopa is commonly used to treat Parkinson's; however, it typically is only therapeutic for approximately five years, after which time the symptoms become aggravated and the use of the drug is stopped.

Some in vitro (test-tube) studies, cell-culture studies (cells growing in petri dishes), and animal studies suggest that supplementation with a single antioxidant may be useful in reducing Parkinson's risk and progression somewhat; however, the effectiveness of individual antioxidants on the risk of developing Parkinson's disease varies, depending on the type of antioxidant, cell type, and assay criteria. Studies with individual antioxidants of Parkinson's in humans have produced inconsistent results, varying from no effect to minimal beneficial effects. The use of one or two dietary or endogenous antioxidants is unlikely to increase the levels of all antioxidant enzymes and dietary and endogenous antioxidants necessary for optimally reducing oxidative stress and chronic inflammation.

This chapter describes studies done with antioxidants, vitamins, and certain herbs in experimental models and human cases of Parkinson's disease. This includes test-tube, cellular, and animal studies. This chapter also presents data and scientific rationale for using a preparation of micronutrients containing multiple dietary and endogenous antioxidants and certain polyphenolic compounds for reducing oxidative stress and chronic inflammation. This preparation of micronutrients may prevent the development of Parkinson's in high-risk populations. The same micronutrient preparation in combination with standard therapy may improve the management of this disease more than is produced by standard therapy alone.

PREVENTION

In Vitro and Animal Model Studies of Vitamins, Antioxidants, and Phenolic Compounds

In Vitro and Cell-Culture Studies

Alpha-synuclein fibrils (in the insoluble aggregated form) are considered toxic to DA neurons. It has been reported that certain antioxidants such as vitamin A, beta-carotene, and coenzyme Q10 inhibited the formation of alpha-synuclein fibrils in a dose-dependent manner, whereas vitamin B_2, vitamin B_6, vitamin C, and vitamin E were ineffective in vitro (Ono and Yamada 2007). In addition, vitamin A, beta-carotene, and coenzyme Q10 destabilized preformed alpha-synuclein fibrils in a dose-dependent manner.

The results of these studies suggest that supplementation with these antioxidants has the potential to reduce the risk of developing Parkinson's by preventing the aggregation of alpha-synuclein and by destabilizing the preformed alpha-synuclein fibrils.

The cellular model of Parkinson's disease can be produced by treating nerve cells with a chemical rotenone, which causes defects in the mitochondria and increases oxidative stress and the accumulation of alpha-synuclein. In a cellular model, pretreatment with B vitamins for a period of four weeks prevented rotenone-induced mitochondrial dysfunction, oxidative stress, and the accumulation of alpha-synuclein (Jia et al. 2010).

Treatment of human nerve cells in culture with a high dose of nicotinamide (a form of vitamin B_3) protected from MPP+-induced cellular toxicity and caused a decrease in complex I and alpha-ketoglutarate dehydrogenase activities, an increase in reactive oxygen species, and oxidation of DNA and protein (Jia et al. 2008).

These studies also revealed that the presence of B vitamins in a micronutrient preparation is essential for producing an optimal beneficial effect in reducing the risk of developing Parkinson's and slowing its progression.

Nicotinamide (vitamin B_3), a precursor of nicotinamide adenine dinucleotide (NAD+), also attenuated glutamate-induced toxicity and preserved cellular levels of NAD+ to support the activity of silent information regulator 1 (SIRT1), a regulator of mitochondrial formation (Liu, Pitta, and Mattson 2008).

This vitamin inhibits oxidative damage and improves mitochondrial function and thus can protect from a degeneration of nerve cells and improve motor function. In addition, in the *Drosophila melanogaster* (fruit fly) model of Parkinson's (an alpha-synuclein transgenic fly), nicotinamide treatment significantly improved motor function (the climbing ability of the fruit fly) (Jia et al. 2008). These studies also revealed that the presence of B vitamins in *any* preparation of multiple antioxidants is essential for producing consistent beneficial effects in experimental models.

Dopamine (DA) is known to induce apoptosis (cell death) in some nerve cells in culture by increasing oxidative stress. The viability of DA-treated human skin melanocytes significantly decreased in a dose-dependent manner, whereas skin keratinocytes exhibited less sensitivity to DA treatment. Treatment with n-acetylcysteine (NAC) or glutathione protected normal human melanocytes from DA-induced toxicity, whereas treatment with other antioxidants, such as vitamin C, vitamin E, trolox, or quercetin, was ineffective (Park et al. 2007).

Auto-oxidation of DA produces excessive amounts of free radicals. Melatonin, deprenyl, and vitamin E inhibited auto-oxidation of DA in a dose-dependent manner, whereas vitamin C was ineffective (Khaldy et al. 2000).

These studies suggest that different antioxidants have different modes of action in protecting skin cells (melanocytes and keratinocytes) against oxidative damage. They further confirmed that only certain antioxidants can protect DA neurons against free radicals generated by the auto-oxidation of DA.

As we have established, the excitatory neurotransmitter glutamate in excessive amounts is toxic to DA neurons by causing increased oxidative stress. This is supported by the fact that the toxic effect of glutamate on DA neurons can be blocked by an analog of NAC (n-acetylcysteine amide) (Penugonda et al. 2005), vitamin E (Schubert, Kimura, and Maher 1992), and coenzyme Q10 (Sandhu et al. 2003).

Animal Models with Vitamin E

6-hydroxydopamine (6-OHDA) and 1-methyl-4-phenyl, 1,2,3,6 tetra-hydropyridine (MPTP) both induced some neurological abnormalities in rodents similar to those observed in human Parkinson's disease. Therefore, these chemicals have been used to evaluate the effectiveness of individual antioxidants in reducing Parkinson's behavior and characteristic neurological abnormalities. Pretreatment of rats with d-alpha-tocopherol or dl-alpha-tocopherol significantly reduced 6-OHDA-induced behavior and biochemical abnormalities (Heim et al. 2001).

Intramuscular administration of d-alpha-tocopheryl succinate, the most effective form of vitamin E (Prasad et al. 2003), protected the 6-OHDA-induced death of DA neurons as well as behavioral and biochemical defects in rats (Pasbakhsh et al. 2008).

Animal Models with Melatonin and Deprenyl

Melatonin secreted by the pineal gland is considered essential for sleep. However, it also exhibits antioxidant activity. Deprenyl, an inhibitor of monoamine oxidase-B (MAO-B), is used in the treatment of early-phase Parkinson's. Melatonin and deprenyl prevent auto-oxidation of DA in a synergistic manner. Melatonin, but not deprenyl treatment, prevented MPTP-induced mitochondrial dysfunction and oxidative damage in DA neurons (Khaldy et al. 2003).

Deprenyl treatment significantly restored an MPTP-induced decrease in DA levels and tyrosine hydroxylase activity; however, the combination of melatonin and deprenyl was more effective than the individual agents (Khaldy et al. 2003).

Animal Models with Antioxidants

Quinolinic acid is an agonist of NMDA receptors and acts like glutamate in causing damage to the nerve cells, whereas 3-nitropropionic acid produces mitochondrial dysfunction. These two chemicals induced oxidative damage and behavioral alterations in animals similar to those observed in Parkinson's patients. The administration of L-carnitine at micromolar (very small) concentrations reduced oxidative damage and behavior abnormalities produced by quinolinic acid or 3-nitropropionic acid (Silva-Adaya et al. 2008).

Some studies revealed that treatment with L-carnitine, coenzyme Q10, alpha-lipoic acid, vitamin E, or resveratrol reduced damage to neurons induced by diverse groups of neurotoxins, such as MPTP, rotenone, and 3-nitropropionic acid (Virmani, Gaetani, and Binienda 2005).

Resveratrol, an activator of SIRT1, stimulates mitochondrial biogenesis in mice and reduces the production of reactive oxygen species (Guarente 2007).

In contrast to SIRT1, SIRT2 promotes the formation of alpha-synuclein fibrils, which are toxic to nerve cells. Inhibitors of SIRT2 prevented the formation of alpha-synuclein fibrils, which are toxic to DA neurons. Inhibitors of SIRT2 also protected DA neurons from chemically induced death and improved symptoms in a *Drosophila melanogaster* (fruit fly) model of Parkinson's disease (Garske, Smith, and Denu 2007).

Therefore, it was suggested that inhibitors of SIRT2 could be useful in treating Parkinson's (Alcain and Villalba 2009).

It has been demonstrated that the treatment of mice with MPTP increased the activity of COX-2 enzyme (which produces inflammation) and lipid peroxides (a marker of oxidative damage) in the homogenates of the midbrain; however, pretreatment with fish oil, melatonin, or vitamin E decreased the levels of these biochemical defects. Treatment with fish oil was more effective in reducing an MPTP-induced rise in COX-2 activity than vitamin E or melatonin, whereas melatonin was more effective in reducing an MPTP-induced rise in lipid peroxides than fish oil or vitamin E (Ortiz et al. 2013).

These results suggest that different antioxidants affect markers of increased oxidative stress and chronic inflammation differently.

Animal Models with Ginkgo Biloba Extract 761

This leaf extract is a patented product comprised of 24 percent flavonoids and 6 percent terpenoids. It has been demonstrated that administration of *Ginkgo biloba* extract 761 in an animal model of Parkinson's protected DA neurons in the midbrain against oxidative damage (Rojas et al. 2012).

Animal Models with Curcumin and a Mixture of Dietary and Endogenous Antioxidants

In collaboration with Dr. Clive Charlton of Meharry Medical College, Nashville, Tennessee, we have found that treatment with curcumin or a mixture of dietary and endogenous antioxidants (a gift from Premier Micronutrient Corporation, Nashville, Tennessee) reduced the incidence of death and hypokinesia that was induced by treating mice with MPTP. Although both curcumin and this antioxidant mixture markedly blocked MPTP-induced depletion of tyrosine hydroxylase (TH) activity, only the antioxidant mixture enhanced the TH activity. This suggests that an antioxidant mixture treatment was more effective than the curcumin treatment in reducing the adverse effects of MPTP in mice.

Animal Models with Black and Green Tea Extract

Black tea extract, which exhibited antioxidant activity, also reduced 6-OHDA-induced degeneration of DA neurons and improved motor and neurochemical deficits (Chaturvedi et al. 2006). A green tea phenolic compound, epigallocatechin-3-gallate, which exhibits antioxidant properties, reduced MPTP-induced Parkinson's in mice through the inhibition of nitric oxide synthase activity (Choi et al. 2002). Increased production of nitric oxide by nitric oxide synthase may increase the levels of peroxynitrite, a highly toxic form of free radical.

HUMAN STUDIES OF VITAMINS, ANTIOXIDANTS, AND PHENOLIC COMPOUNDS ON THE PREVENTION AND PROGRESSION OF PARKINSON'S DISEASE

Human Trials with Vitamin E and Deprenyl

Most clinical trials utilized a single antioxidant, primarily vitamin E (dl-tocopherol). The use of only one antioxidant may have contributed to the inconsistent results obtained in these trials. For example, the effects of deprenyl and tocopherol antioxidative therapy on Parkinson's disease (DATATOP) in a randomized, double-blind, placebo-controlled, multicenter clinical trial was initiated in 1989 to evaluate the efficacy of deprenyl (10 milligrams per day) and dl-tocopherol (2,000 IU per day) individually and in combination in patients with early-stage Parkinson's when no dopa therapy was required. The primary outcome was a prolongation of the time needed for levodopa therapy. After a follow-up period of 8.2 years, deprenyl significantly delayed the time when levodopa therapy was needed, but dl-alpha-tocopherol was ineffective in delaying the time needed for levodopa therapy (Shoulson 1998; Parkinson's Study Group 1993).

There were several flaws in selecting the antioxidant for this study, which are described here. The use of a single dietary antioxidant vitamin E was one major flaw in this study design in view of the fact that glutathione deficiency in the brain is a consistent finding in most neurodegenerative diseases, including Parkinson's. Therefore, the addition of a glutathione-elevating agent such as alpha-lipoic acid and n-acetylcysteine would have been useful. Mitochondrial dysfunction is also commonly observed in Parkinson's; therefore, the addition of coenzyme Q10 and L-carnitine, which improve the function of mitochondria, would have been useful in producing beneficial effects on its symptoms.

There was another flaw in the DATATOP study design, pertaining to an antioxidant. A multiple vitamin preparation was allowed for all individuals who wished to take it. It was argued that the effects of the 30 IU of vitamin E present in the multiple vitamin preparation would not significantly contribute to the effects of 2,000 IU of vitamin E. This argument may not be valid, given that antioxidants in a multiple vitamin preparation interact with each other in a synergistic manner in producing biological effects (Prasad and Kumar 1996). Therefore, the impact of 30 IU of vitamin E administered in a multiple vitamin preparation would be more pronounced than that produced by 30 IU of vitamin E alone. Hence, the consumption of a multiple vitamin preparation containing a low dose of vitamin E by control subjects is likely to create an unacceptable variable while evaluating the efficacy of high-dose vitamin E alone in early Parkinson's patients. This is particularly true given that both the experimental group and the placebo group were permitted to take a multiple vitamin preparation in an uncontrolled fashion—no effort was made to track which individuals took the multiple vitamins or their possible effects.

As we have determined—and articulated in other areas of this book but which bears repeating here—patients with Parkinson's have a high oxidative environment in the brain. It is known that individual antioxidants, when oxidized, act as prooxidants. This may compromise the effectiveness of the antioxidant. Furthermore, the use of a single antioxidant may not increase the levels of all antioxidant enzymes and dietary and endogenous antioxidants necessary for optimally reducing oxidative stress and chronic inflammation. Therefore, the conclusion of the DATATOP study—that antioxidants are not useful in reducing the progression of Parkinson's—is not valid.

Vitamin E and Humans: An Epidemiologic Study

Some epidemiologic studies suggest that a diet rich in vitamin E may reduce the risk of Parkinson's disease (Zhang et al. 2002; Etminan, Gill, and Samii 2005). The results of these epidemiologic studies with vitamin E conflict with the results obtained from intervention trials. It's possible that in the studies cited above the diet of the individuals studied contained antioxidants other than vitamin E; therefore, its interaction with other antioxidants may have contributed to the beneficial effect of reducing the risk. Thus, epidemiologic studies would favor the use of multiple antioxidants in any clinical Parkinson's study.

Human Trials with Coenzyme Q10

In a multicenter, randomized, double-blind, placebo-controlled trial on 80 early-stage Parkinson's patients who did not require any therapy, the efficacy of coenzyme Q10 at doses of 300, 600, or 1,200 milligrams per day was evaluated. The primary outcome was the development of the Unified Parkinson's Disease Rating Score (UPDRS), and the patients were followed for 16 months, or until disability, which required levodopa therapy, was needed. The results showed that coenzyme Q10 at the highest dose of 1,200 milligrams per day was safe and well tolerated by patients. The results also revealed that less disability developed in patients receiving coenzyme Q10 compared to placebo controls; the benefit was greater in patients receiving the highest dosage (Shults et al. 2002).

Reviews of several open and controlled clinical studies revealed that daily supplementation with coenzyme Q10 either had no effect or had minimal benefit in early-stage Parkinson's patients (Weber and Ernst 2006; Storch et al. 2007).

Trials Lacking for NAD/NADH

No studies have been performed with nicotinamide adenine dinucleotide (NAD) or nicotinamide (vitamin B_3), a precursor of NAD in human Parkinson's.

Human Trials with Vitamin E and Vitamin C in Combination with Anti-Cholinergic Drugs

In an open-labeled clinical trial, the efficacy of high doses of alpha-tocopherol and ascorbate was tested in early-stage Parkinson's patients. Patients were allowed to receive amantadine (which increases dopamine release and prevents the reuptake of dopamine) and an anti-cholinergic drug, but not levodopa or a DA agonist. The primary outcome was a delay of the time that levodopa therapy was needed by 2.5 years (Fahn 1992). This study shows that in patients with early-stage disease a mixture of antioxidants—rather than a single antioxidant—may be a better approach in delaying the time when levodopa therapy is needed.

MANAGEMENT STRATEGIES
How to Reduce Oxidative Stress and Chronic Inflammation, Relevant Studies

Significant studies discussed in this chapter suggest that increased oxidative stress and chronic inflammation play an important role in the development and progression of Parkinson's disease in humans. Therefore, it's essential to develop a formulation of micronutrients that can optimally reduce oxidative stress and chronic inflammation.

Reducing Oxidative Stress

Oxidative stress in the body occurs when the antioxidant system fails to provide adequate protection against damage caused by free radicals (reactive oxygen species and reactive nitrogen species). Increased oxidative stress in the body can be reduced most effectively by elevating the levels of antioxidant enzymes as well as dietary and endogenous antioxidant chemicals, because they work in part by different mechanisms. For example, antioxidant enzymes reduce free radicals by catalysis (converting free radicals to nontoxic compounds), whereas dietary and endogenous antioxidant chemicals reduce free radicals by directly scavenging them.

Normally, in response to increased reactive oxygen species (ROS), Nrf2 (nuclear factor-erythroid 2-related factor 2), a form of protein, is activated. When Nrf2 is activated, it translocates from the cytoplasm to the nucleus, where it binds with ARE (antioxidant response element), which increases the levels of antioxidant enzymes and detoxifying enzymes in order to reduce oxidative damage (Itoh et al. 1997; Hayes et al. 2000; Chan, Han, and Kan 2001). In response to increased oxidative stress, existing levels of dietary and endogenous antioxidant chemicals also participate in decreasing oxidative stress, resulting in reduced levels of these antioxidants in the body. The levels of dietary and endogenous antioxidants cannot be elevated without supplementation.

Factors Regulating Response of Nrf2 and Its Action

Several studies suggest that antioxidant enzymes are elevated by Nrf2 activation, which depends on ROS-dependent (Niture et al. 2010) and ROS-independent mechanisms (Xi et al. 2012; Li et al. 2012; Bergstrom et al. 2011; Wruck et al. 2008; Hine and Mitchell 2012). In addition, the levels of antioxidant enzymes are also dependent on the binding ability of Nrf2 with ARE in the nucleus (Suh et al. 2004).

Differential Response of Nrf2 to ROS Generated During Acute and Chronic Oxidative Stress

Excessive amounts of ROS are generated during acute oxidative stress, which occurs during strenuous exercise, for example. Increased levels of ROS are also present during chronic oxidative stress, which occurs with Parkinson's disease. It appears that Nrf2 responds to ROS generated during acute and chronic oxidative stress differently. During acute transient oxidative stress Nrf2 responds to ROS and translocates itself from the cytoplasm to the nucleus, where it binds with ARE to increase the expression of antioxidant genes, which then produce increased levels of antioxidant enzymes. This response of Nrf2 to ROS protects neurons from the damage produced by ROS.

The fact that increased levels of chronic oxidative stress are found in Parkinson's patients suggests that the Nrf2-ARE pathway responsible for increasing the levels of antioxidant enzymes has become unresponsive to ROS in this disease.

Age-related decline in antioxidant enzymes in the livers of older rats compared to that of younger rats was due to a reduction in the binding ability of Nrf2 with ARE in the nucleus. However, treatment with alpha-lipoic acid restored this defect, increased the levels of antioxidant enzymes, and restored the loss of glutathione from the livers of old rats (Suh et al. 2004). The exact reasons for the Nrf2-ARE regulatory system to become unresponsive to ROS during chronic oxidative stress are unknown; however, defects in the binding ability of Nrf2 with ARE may be one of the possible reasons.

Nrf2 in Parkinson's Disease

The levels of Nrf2 in the nucleus decreased in the hippocampal neurons of Parkinson's patients despite increased oxidative stress (Ramsey et al. 2007). This suggests that the Nrf2-ARE pathway becomes unresponsive to ROS stimulation, resulting in reduced translocation from the cytoplasm to the nucleus. It is also possible that Nrf2's binding ability with ARE is impaired. It's not known whether the defect in the Nrf2 pathway occurs in the cytoplasm, where Nrf2 forms a complex with Keap-1 (an inhibitor of Nrf2), or at the level of the nucleus, where it binds with ARE to enhance the expression of antioxidant genes—or at both levels.

Treatment with lactacystin, a proteasome inhibitor, reduced 6-hydroxydopamine (6-OHDA)-induced damage to nerve cells by reducing oxidative stress. This protective effect of lactacystin against 6-OHDA-induced toxicity was due to the activation of the Nrf2-ARE pathway (Izumi 2013). The same author isolated a new activator of Nrf2 from the green perilla leaves—2-3-dihydroxy-4-6-dimethoxychalcone (DDC)—which protected nerve cells against the toxicity of 6-OHDA.

Treatment with naringenin, a natural flavonoid compound, protected 6-OHDA-induced damage to nerve cells in culture and in mice by reducing oxidative stress via activating the Nrf2-ARE pathway (Lou et al. 2013).

Oral administration of a synthetic triterpenoid (TP) reduced MPTP-induced damage to DA neurons in mice by reducing oxidative stress via activation of the Nrf2-ARE pathway (Kaidery et al. 2013).

All antioxidants can destroy free radicals to varying degrees; however, some of them can activate Nrf2 by a ROS-independent mechanism, while others can activate Nrf2 by a ROS-dependent mechanism.

Antioxidant compounds that activate Nrf2 by a ROS-independent mechanism: Some examples are vitamin E and genistein (Xi et al. 2012), alpha-lipoic acid (Suh et al. 2004), curcumin (Trujillo et al., 2013), resveratrol (Steele et al. 2013; Kode et al. 2008), omega-3-fatty acids, (Gao et al. 2007; Saw et al. 2013), glutathione (Song et al. 2014), NAC (Ji et al. 2010), and coenzyme Q10 (Choi et al. 2009). Several plant-derived phytochemicals, such as epigallocatechin-3-gallate, carestol, kahweol, cinnamonyl-based compounds, zerumbone, lycopene and carnosol (Chun et al. 2014; Jaramillo et al. 2013; Jeong et al. 2006), allicin, a major organosulfur compound found in garlic (Li et al. 2012), sulforaphane, a organosulfur compound, found in cruciferous vegetables, (Bergstrom et al. 2011), and kavalactones (methysticin, kavain and yangonin) (Wruck et al. 2008). The mechanisms of activation of Nrf2 without ROS stimulation are not known.

Antioxidant compound that activates Nrf2 by a ROS-dependent mechanism: L-carnitine activates Nrf2 without the need for ROS stimulation (Zambrano et al. 2013) probably by generating transient ROS.

Activation of Nrf2 in astrocytes protected reduced mutated alpha-synuclein-induced damage to the nerve cells in mice (Gan et al. 2012).

The DJ-1 gene is responsible for providing protection to the nerve cells against oxidative damage. This protective effect of DJ-1 on the nerve cells was due to activation of the Nrf2-ARE pathway. This is evidenced by the fact that increased levels of DJ-1 cause translocation of Nrf2 from the cytoplasm to the nucleus, where it binds with ARE to increase the levels of antioxidant enzymes (Im et al. 2012).

A combination of selected agents from the above groups may optimally reduce oxidative stress, and thereby may reduce the risk of developing Parkinson's. In combination with standard therapy they may also improve the management of this disease.

Now let's take a look at chronic inflammation and see how a similar application of antioxidants may be helpful here as well.

Reducing Chronic Inflammation

In addition to reducing oxidative stress, some individual antioxidants from the above groups have been shown to reduce chronic inflammation (Abate et al. 2000; Devaraj et al. 2007; Fu et al. 2008; Lee et al. 2007; Peairs and Rankin 2008; Rahman et al. 2008; Suzuki, Aggarwal, and Packer 1992; Zhu et al. 2008). A combination of these antioxidants may optimally reduce chronic inflammation and therefore may reduce the risk of developing Parkinson's disease and, in combination with standard therapy, may improve the management of this disease. (These same antioxidants are also beneficial in the case of Huntington's disease, which we will explore in greater detail in chapter 7.)

PROBLEMS OF USING A SINGLE ANTIOXIDANT IN PARKINSON'S DISEASE

Laboratory studies consistently showed that supplementation with individual antioxidants such as vitamin A, beta-carotene, vitamin C, vitamin E, coenzyme Q10, n-acetylcysteine, alpha-lipoic acid, L-carnitine, resveratrol, curcumin, B vitamins, and omega-3 fatty acids reduced the symptoms and improved neurochemical changes in Parkinson's animal models. And although epidemiologic studies revealed that a diet rich in vitamin E may reduce the risk, clinical trials with an individual antioxidant have been inconsistent, producing minimal benefits at best.

In Parkinson's patients the levels of oxidative stress are elevated in the brain. Administration of a single antioxidant in such patients may not be effective, because this antioxidant may be oxidized in the presence of a high oxidative environment and then act as a prooxidant. In addition, the dose requirement of a single antioxidant—in producing any beneficial effect in patients—may be so high that it can cause toxicity following long-term consumption.

Previous studies associated with other chronic diseases, such as beta-carotene in male smokers, whose use of tobacco is considered heavy, for reducing the risk of lung cancer; vitamin E in Alzheimer's disease for improving cognitive function; and vitamin E in Parkinson's disease for improving symptoms of the disease, as expected, produced inconsistent results. These inconsistent results varied from no effect with Parkinson's (Shoulson 1998) to modest beneficial (Sano et al. 1997) or no effect with Alzheimer's disease (Farina et al. 2012), and harmful effects with male smokers (Albanes et al. 1995). It is not possible to optimally reduce oxidative stress and chronic inflammation by the use of one or two antioxidants in Parkinson's patients, because they may not increase the levels of antioxidant enzymes as well as dietary and endogenous antioxidants in the body.

Thus I recommend a preparation of micronutrients containing multiple dietary and endogenous antioxidants, B vitamins, vitamin D, certain minerals, polyphenolic compounds (resveratrol, curcumin), and omega-3 fatty acids for reducing the risk of developing Parkinson's and for improving the effectiveness of standard therapy in its management.

RATIONALE FOR USING MULTIPLE ANTIOXIDANTS IN PARKINSON'S DISEASE*

The mechanisms of action of antioxidants in the proposed formulation are in part different. Their distribution in various organs and cells, their affinity with various types of free radicals, and their biological half-lives are different. For example, beta-carotene (BC) is more effective in scavenging oxygen radicals than most other antioxidants. Beta-carotene can perform certain biological functions that cannot be produced by vitamin A, and vitamin A can perform certain biological functions that cannot be performed by beta-carotene. It has been reported that BC treatment enhances the expression of the connexin gene, which codes for a gap junction protein in mammalian fibroblasts in culture, whereas vitamin A treatment does not produce such an effect. Vitamin A can induce differentiation in certain normal cells and cancer cells, whereas BC and other carotenoids do not. Thus, BC and vitamin A have, in part, different functions in the body.

The gradient of oxygen pressure varies within the cells. Some antioxidants such as vitamin E are more effective as scavengers of free radicals in an environment featuring reduced oxygen pressure, whereas BC and vitamin A are more effective in environments featuring a higher atmospheric pressure.

Cells contain mostly water and some fat. Cellular components are distributed in the water and fat of the cells. Vitamin C is necessary to protect cellular components in the water portion of the cells, whereas carotenoids, vitamin A, and vitamin E protect cellular components in the fat portion of the cells. Vitamin C also plays an important role in maintaining cellular levels of vitamin E by recycling the oxidized form of vitamin E, which acts as a prooxidant, to the reduced form of vitamin E, which acts as an antioxidant.

---

*The references for this section are described in a review (Prasad, Cole, and Prasad 2002).

The *form* of vitamin E used is also important in a micronutrient preparation. It has been established that d-alpha-tocopheryl succinate (vitamin E succinate) is the most effective form of vitamin E both in vitro and in vivo. This form of vitamin E is more soluble than alpha-tocopherol and enters cells more readily. Therefore, it is expected to cross the blood-brain barrier in greater amounts than alpha-tocopherol does.

We have reported that an oral ingestion of alpha-tocopheryl succinate (800 IU per day) in humans increased the plasma levels not only of alpha-tocopherol but also of vitamin E succinate. This suggests that a portion of vitamin E succinate can be absorbed from the intestinal tract before conversion to alpha-tocopherol. This observation is important, because the conventional assumption based on studies in rodents has been that esterified forms of vitamin E such as alpha-tocopheryl succinate, alpha-tocopheryl nicotinate, and alpha-tocopheryl acetate can be absorbed from the intestinal tract only after they are converted to the alpha-tocopherol form. Our preliminary data showed that this assumption may not be true for absorption of vitamin E succinate in humans, provided the pool of alpha-tocopherol in the blood is saturated.

The endogenous antioxidant glutathione is effective in destroying H_2O_2 and superoxide anion (a form of free radical). However, oral supplementation with glutathione failed to significantly increase the plasma levels of glutathione in humans, suggesting that glutathione is completely destroyed in the intestine. Therefore, I propose to utilize n-acetylcysteine (NAC) and alpha-lipoic acid, which increase the cellular levels of glutathione by different mechanisms in a micronutrient preparation.

Coenzyme Q10 is another endogenous antioxidant that may have some potential value in the prevention and improved treatment of Parkinson's disease. Coenzyme Q10 administration has been shown to improve some clinical symptoms in Parkinson's patients (Shults et al. 2002). Given that mitochondrial dysfunction is associated with the disease and because coenzyme Q10 is needed for the generation of ATP by mitochondria, it is essential to add this antioxidant to a micronutrient preparation. A study has shown that coenzyme Q10 scavenges peroxy radicals faster than alpha-tocopherol and, like vitamin C, can convert oxidized vitamin E to a reduced form of vitamin E, which acts as an antioxidant.

Nicotinamide (vitamin B$_3$) attenuated glutamate-induced toxicity in nerve cells. Nicotinamide is also an inhibitor of histone deacetylase activity and has restored memory deficits in other neurodegenerative diseases such as is found in Alzheimer's diseased transgenic mice. These preclinical data suggest that oral supplementation with nicotinamide may be safe and useful in the prevention and improved treatment of Parkinson's. Selenium is a cofactor of glutathione peroxidase, and Se-glutathione peroxidase acts as an antioxidant by increasing the intracellular level of glutathione.

In addition to dietary and endogenous antioxidants, B vitamins, especially high doses of vitamin B$_3$ (nicotinamide), should be added to a multiple micronutrient preparation. B vitamins are also essential for normal brain function. Omega-3 fatty acids were also added, because a few studies of animal models show some benefits.

Two recent clinical studies showed that supplementation with multiple vitamin preparations reduced cancer incidence by 10 percent in men (Gaziano et al. 2012) and improved clinical outcomes in patients with HIV/AIDS who were not taking medication (Baum et al. 2013).

RATIONALE FOR USING AN NSAID IN PREVENTION OF PARKINSON'S DISEASE

Inflammatory reactions represent one of the major factors that initiate and promote the degeneration of DA neurons in the Parkinson's brain. Thus, the use of an NSAID in the prevention and treatment of Parkinson's appears rational. Laboratory data have shown that products of inflammatory reactions such as prostaglandins (Prasad, La Rosa, and Prasad 1998), cytokines (Shalit et al. 1994), complement proteins

(Rogers et al. 1995), adhesion molecules (Verbeek et al. 1994), and free radicals (Smith et al. 1995) are neurotoxic. Thus, the use of low-dose aspirin (81 milligrams per day) to prevent and reduce the Parkinson's progression remains a viable option.

CAN FAMILIAL PARKINSON'S BE PREVENTED OR DELAYED?

It's often believed that familial Parkinson's disease (a family history of the disease) cannot be prevented or delayed by any pharmacological and/or physiological means. Laboratory experiments on the genetic basis of another disease model (cancer) in the *Drosophila melanogaster* (fruit fly) show that it may be possible to prevent or at least delay the onset of the familial basis of Parkinson's.

The gene HOP (TUM-1) is essential to the development of fruit flies. A mutation in this gene markedly increases the risk of developing a leukemia-like tumor in female flies (unpublished observation in collaboration with Dr. Bhattacharya et al. of NASA, Moffat Field, California). Proton radiation is a powerful cancer-causing agent. Whole-body irradiation with proton radiation dramatically increased the incidence of cancer in these irradiated flies compared to that of unirradiated flies.

The question arose as to whether a preparation of multiple antioxidants can reduce the incidence of cancer that is due to a specific gene defect. To test this possibility a mixture of multiple dietary and endogenous antioxidants were fed to these flies through the diet seven days before proton irradiation and was continued throughout the experimental period of seven days.

The results showed that antioxidant treatment before and after irradiation totally blocked the proton radiation-induced cancer in fruit flies. This finding on fruit flies is of particular interest, because, to my knowledge, this is the first demonstration in which the genetic basis of a disease can be prevented by supplementation with multiple antioxidants. This observation made on fruit flies cannot be readily extrapolated to humans, however, and it is unknown whether daily supplementation with multiple antioxidants in children of parents who have a family history of Parkinson's can prevent or delay the onset of the disease. The results on fruit flies, however, do suggest that daily supplementation with multiple antioxidants could potentially prevent or delay the onset of symptoms for those individuals with a family history. A clinical study to test the effectiveness of the proposed strategies among those who have a family history should be tested.

Before discussing the strategies for prevention, it's essential to define primary and secondary prevention. The purpose of primary prevention is to protect healthy individuals, such as individuals fifty years of age or older and individuals with a family history of Parkinson's, from developing this disease. The purpose of secondary prevention is to stop or slow the progression in individuals who exhibit early signs but are not taking any medication.

PRIMARY PREVENTION OF PARKINSON'S DISEASE IN HUMANS

To develop primary prevention strategies, it's essential to identify external risk factors that increase the risk of developing Parkinson's disease. Some human epidemiologic studies have identified environment- and lifestyle-related agents that increase the risk of developing it. These agents include exposure to manganese (Mn), pesticides, herbicides, the designer drug meperidene, and certain solvents such as trichloroethylene (TCE), perchloroethylene (PERC), and carbon tetrachloride (CCl). For primary prevention I would suggest that exposure to the above agents should be avoided. And as mentioned earlier in chapter 4, although epidemiologic studies suggest that cigarette smoking reduces the risk, I would not recommend it because of the other serious adverse consequences it engenders.

Given that increased oxidative stress and chronic inflammation play a role in the development of Parkinson's, it would be essential to utilize a preparation of micronutrients that can reduce oxidative stress and chronic inflammation by elevating antioxidant enzymes as well as dietary and endogenous antioxidants for primary prevention. The ingredients and their doses are listed in table 5.1 on page 108.

RECOMMENDED MICRONUTRIENTS
IN COMBINATION WITH LOW-DOSE ASPIRIN
FOR THE PRIMARY PREVENTION
OF PARKINSON'S DISEASE

Individuals with a family history of Parkinson's and those age fifty or older are very suitable candidates for investigating the effectiveness of the proposed micronutrients in combination with a low-dose aspirin for primary prevention. The selected combination of nontoxic agents includes vitamin A (retinyl palmitate), vitamin E (both d-alpha-tocopherol and d-alpha-tocopheryl succinate), natural mixed carotenoids, vitamin C (calcium ascorbate), B vitamins with higher levels of vitamin B_3 (nicotinamide), vitamin D, selenium, coenzyme Q10, alpha-lipoic acid, n-acetylcysteine (NAC), L-carnitine, omega-3 fatty acids, resveratrol, and curcumin. The combination of above agents was selected because they are capable of optimally reducing oxidative stress and chronic inflammation by activating the Nrf2-ARE pathway without ROS stimulation and by directly scavenging free radicals. The daily doses can be divided in two (with half taken in the morning and half in the evening, preferably with a meal). Below is further explanation of different components of the suggested regimen.

Uniqueness of the proposed formulation of micronutrients: The proposed formulation of micronutrients has no iron, copper, manganese, or heavy metals (vanadium, zirconium, or molybdenum). Iron and copper were not added, because they're known to interact with vitamin C and generate excessive amounts of free radicals. In addition, iron and copper are absorbed more in the presence of antioxidants than in the absence of antioxidants. Therefore, it's possible that prolonged consumption of these trace minerals in the presence of antioxidants may increase the levels of free iron or copper stores in the body, because there are no significant mechanisms of excretion of iron among men of all ages and women after menopause.

Increased stores of free iron or copper may increase the risk of some human chronic diseases including Parkinson's disease. Increased iron stores have been linked to increased risk of several chronic diseases including Parkinson's (Olanow and Arendash 1994). Heavy metals were not added, because prolonged consumption of these metals may increase their levels in the body due to the fact that there is no significant mechanism of excretion of these metals from the body. High levels of these metals are considered neurotoxic. The effectiveness of the proposed micronutrient preparation and a low-dose aspirin for high-risk populations, such as individuals fifty or older and individuals with a family history, should be tested by a well-designed clinical study.

Dose-schedule: Most clinical studies with antioxidants in Parkinson's disease have utilized a once-a-day dose schedule. Taking vitamins and antioxidants once a day, however, can create large fluctuations of their levels in the body. This is due to the fact that the biological half-lives of vitamins and antioxidants vary markedly depending on their lipid or water solubility. A twofold difference in the levels of vitamin E succinate can produce marked alterations in the expression profiles of several genes in nerve cells in culture. Therefore, taking a multiple vitamin preparation once a day may produce large fluctuations in the levels of micronutrients in the body, which could potentially cause genetic stress in the cells. This may compromise the effectiveness of the vitamin supplementation after long-term consumption.

I recommend taking the proposed preparation of micronutrients twice a day to reduce fluctuation of the levels of gene expressions in the body. Such a dose schedule may improve the effectiveness of the proposed micronutrient preparation in reducing the development of the disease.

Toxicity of antioxidants present in the proposed micronutrient preparation: Antioxidants, B vitamins, and certain polyphenolic compounds (curcumin and resveratrol) used in the proposed micronutrient preparation are considered safe. Antioxidants at doses higher than those recommended for the proposed micronutrient preparation have been consumed by the U.S. population for decades without significant toxicity. However, a few of them may produce harmful effects at certain high doses in some individuals when consumed daily for a long period of time. For example, vitamin A at doses of 10,000 IU or more per day can cause birth defects in pregnant women, and beta-carotene at doses of 50 milligrams or more can produce bronzing of the skin that's reversible on discontinuation. Vitamin C as ascorbic acid at high doses (10 grams or more per day) can cause diarrhea in some individuals. Vitamin E at high doses (2,000 IU or more per day) can induce clotting defects after long-term consumption. Vitamin B_6 at high doses (50 milligrams or more per day) may produce peripheral neuropathy, and selenium at doses of 400 micrograms or more per day can cause skin and liver toxicity after long-term use. Coenzyme Q10 has no known toxicity; recommended daily doses are 30 to 400 milligrams. N-acetylcysteine (NAC) doses of 250 to 1,500 milligrams and alpha-lipoic acid doses of 600 milligrams are used in humans without toxicity at these doses. All ingredients present in the proposed micronutrient preparations are safe and are classified as food supplements; therefore, they don't require FDA approval for their use.

Aspirin: A low-dose aspirin is recommended because of its anti-inflammatory effect, and because, in combination with vitamin E, it produced a synergistic effect on the inhibition of cyclooxygenase activity (Abate et al. 2000). Therefore, the combination of these two agents (a low-dose aspirin and vitamin E) may be more effective in reducing the levels of chronic inflammation than the individual agents. A low-dose aspirin (81 milligrams per day) is recommended by cardiologists to reduce the risk of heart disease; however, it can cause intestinal bleeding in some individuals after long-term consumption.

RECOMMENDATIONS FOR SECONDARY PREVENTION OF PARKINSON'S DISEASE IN HUMANS

Reducing exposure to the external risk factors detailed in the discussion about primary prevention is also relevant for secondary prevention. Reduction of oxidative stress and chronic inflammation by the same preparation of micronutrients is equally important for secondary prevention.

The strategies proposed for primary prevention may also be used for secondary prevention in patients with early-phase Parkinson's who are not taking any medications. A clinical study to test the effectiveness of the proposed strategies in reducing the disease's progression should be initiated.

TREATMENT OF PARKINSON'S DISEASE IN HUMANS

The purpose of treatment is to slow the progression of disease and improve its symptoms. Specifically, the purpose of drug treatment is to increase the functioning of surviving dopamine (DA) neurons by maintaining adequate levels of DA in the brain. To accomplish this, L-dopa (levodopa), a precursor of DA and DA receptor agonists, is used. Deprenyl (monoamine oxidase inhibitor) and catechol-o-methyl transferase (COMT) inhibitor are also used to prevent the degradation of DA. In addition, in some cases an acetylcholinesterase inhibitor is utilized to balance the two neurotransmitters—DA and acetylcholine—by reducing the levels of acetylcholine. None of the treatment with drugs or surgery inhibits oxidative stress and chronic inflammation; therefore, DA neurons continue to die despite these treatments.

Although medication and surgery offer relief for those persons afflicted with Parkinson's disease, there is currently no known cure for the disease. Often the levodopa utilized to treat the symptoms of Parkinson's is combined with carbidopa, because carbidopa helps the levodopa bolster the brain's stores of dopamine, which is essential in treating the disease. The carbidopa does this by helping with the timing mechanism involved with this process.

And although levodopa is helpful to roughly 75 percent of persons with Parkinson's disease, not all symptoms are alleviated with its use. Symptoms that *are* responsive to it include the slow body movements that characterize Parkinson's disease, as well as associated rigidity. Tremor presents more of a challenge, although anticholinergic drugs may help with this particular symptom.

Other drugs used in the treatment include bromocriptine, pramipexole, and ropinirole, which replicate the actions of dopamine in the brain; indeed, the brain's neurons respond to these drugs in the same way that they do to dopamine. Another useful medication in the treatment of Parkinson's is amantadine, an anti-viral. Rasagiline is yet another drug used, typically in advanced patients and in combination with levodopa. Rasagiline is also used alone to treat persons afflicted with early-stage Parkinson's.

For those persons with Parkinson's that are unresponsive to drugs, surgery is an option. Deep brain stimulation (DBS), wherein the brain is wired with electrodes so that an electric current can be used therapeutically on it, has found approval from the U.S. Food and Drug Administration. The use of DBS is advantageous in that not only does it obviate the need for medication, but it also mitigates dyskinesia, the involuntary jerking and twitching motions that frequently are a by-product of the medications used to treat the disease. DBS may also alleviate some of the other symptoms; however, the technology requires careful programming for the stimulator device to work in the most optimal fashion (see www.ninds.nih.gov/disorders/parkinsons_disease/parkinsons_disease.htm).

PROPOSED MICRONUTRIENT SUPPLEMENT AND LOW-DOSES OF NSAID IN COMBINATION WITH STANDARD THERAPY IN PARKINSON'S PATIENTS

Levodopa therapy is considered the gold standard for the treatment of Parkinson's disease; however, in vitro studies suggest that treatment of neuronal cells in culture with L-dopa is very toxic, thus treatment in humans is discontinued after about five years. This toxic effect is no doubt due to the fact that L-dopa generates excessive amounts of free radicals during auto-oxidation as well as during the oxidative metabolism of its product, DA.

It should also be noted, however, that in animal studies it appears that there is no evidence of similar effects of L-dopa in vivo (Melamed et al. 1998). In a randomized, double-blind, placebo-controlled trial involving 361 patients with early-stage Parkinson's, the effects of various doses of levodopa for a period of forty weeks were investigated (Fahn et al. 2004). The results showed that the patients receiving the highest dose of levodopa had significantly more dyskinesia, hypertonia, infection, headache, and nausea than those receiving placebo. The clinical data showed that levodopa treatment either slowed the progression or improved the symptoms of the disease. However, neuroimaging data suggested that levodopa treatment increased the rate of loss of nigrostriatal DA nerve terminals, or it reduced the levels of DA transporter more than was produced by placebo treatment.

A further investigation of this issue revealed that the dose amount of levodopa is a factor in producing motor complications of dyskinesia, and these can develop as early as five to six months at high levodopa doses (Fahn 2005). Given that levodopa has the potential to cause increased oxidative damage both in the brain and outside the brain, it appears rational to propose that reducing oxidative stress and chronic inflammation in combination with standard therapy may be one of the rational choices for reducing the progression and improving management. Such a strategy may improve the effectiveness of levodopa therapy by reducing the side effects that occur as a result of increased oxidative damage. This would then allow levodopa treatment to be effective for a longer period than is utilized at present and may even allow for a reduction of the dosage of levodopa without sacrificing its efficacy.

WHAT'S IN THE FORMULATION AND HOW MUCH TO TAKE

The formulation of micronutrients proposed for the primary and secondary prevention of Parkinson's disease can also be used in combination with standard therapy and a low-dose aspirin to reduce the progression and improve its management more than that produced by standard therapy alone. The effectiveness of the proposed micronutrient strategy in combination with standard therapy should be tested by well-designed clinical trials. In the meantime, the proposed micronutrient strategy may be adopted by Parkinson's patients who are receiving standard therapy in consultation with their physicians or health care professionals. It is expected that the proposed recommendations would enhance the effectiveness of standard therapy by reducing progression and improving symptoms.

The proposed micronutrient preparation recommended for adults (fifty years or older) is presented in table 5.1 on page 108. Please e-mail knprasad@comcast.net for information regarding products.

TABLE 5.1. INGREDIENTS OF A RECOMMENDED MICRONUTRIENT PREPARATION FOR THE PREVENTION AND IMPROVED MANAGEMENT OF PARKINSON'S DISEASE (DAILY DOSES)*

Vitamin A (retinyl palmitate)	3,000 IU
Natural Vitamin E	400 IU (d-alpha-tocopheryl succinate 300 IU) (d-alpha-tocopheryl acetate 100 IU)
Vitamin C (calcium ascorbate)	1,500 mg
Vitamin D_3 (cholecalciferol)	1,000 IU
Vitamin B_1 (thiamine mononitrate)	4 mg
Vitamin B_2 (riboflavin)	5 mg
Vitamin B_3 (nicotinamide)	200 mg
Vitamin B_6 (pyridoxine hydrochloride)	5 mg
Folic acid	800 mcg
Vitamin B_{12} (cyanocobalamin)	10 mcg
Biotin	200 mcg
Pantothenic acid (calcium pantothenate)	10 mg
Zinc glycinate	15 mg
Selenium (seleno-L-methionine)	200 mcg
Chromium (as picolinate)	50 mcg
N-acetylcysteine (NAC)	proprietary dose†
Coenzyme Q10	proprietary dose
Alpha-lipoic acid	proprietary dose
L-carnitine	proprietary dose
Resveratrol	proprietary dose
Curcumin	proprietary dose
Omega-3 fatty acids	proprietary dose

*Daily doses are divided into two doses, half to be taken in the morning and half in the evening, preferably with a meal. Children age 5–12 with a family history of Parkinson's disease should take 20 percent of the adult dose. Adolescents age 13–17 with a family history of Parkinson's disease should take 40 percent of the adult dose.
†Total amount of proprietary active blend is 1,620 mg.

DIET AND LIFESTYLE RECOMMENDATIONS FOR PARKINSON'S DISEASE

Even though there is no direct link between diet- and lifestyle-related factors and the development or progression of Parkinson's, it's always useful to adhere to a balanced diet that is low in fat and high in fiber, with plenty of fruits and vegetables. In terms of fruit, blueberries and raspberries are particularly important because of their protective role against oxidative injuries in the brain. Lifestyle recommendations include daily moderate exercise, reduced stress, and no tobacco smoking or drug use.

CONCLUDING REMARKS

The results of many studies presented in this review suggest that increased oxidative stress and chronic inflammation play a dominant role in the development and progression of Parkinson's disease. Even in familial Parkinson's, these biochemical defects play a crucial role in the disease's development and progression. Therefore, the optimal reduction of oxidative stress and chronic inflammation appears to be a logical choice in preventing Parkinson's and, in combination with standard therapy, to improve its management. The use of a single antioxidant or certain polyphenolic compound is unlikely to achieve the above goal of reducing oxidative stress and chronic inflammation. Unfortunately, as we have established, most laboratory and clinical studies have been performed with a single antioxidant, producing some beneficial effects in animal models and zero or minimal effects in humans.

Therefore, I have proposed a formulation of micronutrients containing nontoxic agents such as vitamin A (retinyl palmitate), B vitamins—with higher levels of vitamin B_3 (nicotinamide)—vitamin C (calcium ascorbate), vitamin D, vitamin E (both d-alpha-tocopherol and d-alpha-tocopheryl succinate), natural mixed carotenoids, selenium, coenzyme Q10, alpha-lipoic acid, n-acetylcysteine (NAC), L-carnitine, omega-3 fatty acids, resveratrol, and curcumin for primary and secondary prevention. The same formulation of micronutrients in combination with standard therapy may reduce the progression of Parkinson's disease and improve its symptoms more than is produced by standard therapy alone.

This combination of substances was selected because it is capable of optimally reducing oxidative stress and chronic inflammation by activating the Nrf2-ARE pathway without ROS stimulation and by directly scavenging free radicals. Again, no iron, copper, manganese, or heavy metals (vanadium, zirconium, or molybdenum) have been added to the above preparation. The daily doses should be divided in two (half to be taken in the morning and half in the evening, preferably with a meal). One's diet should be low in fat, high in fiber, and contain an abundance of antioxidants. In terms of lifestyle considerations, the lifestyle should feature exercise on a regular daily basis, reduced stress, and no tobacco smoking or drug use.

At present there are no effective strategies for the prevention of Parkinson's disease. Clinical studies using the proposed micronutrient formulation and a low-dose aspirin should be initiated for the primary prevention in high-risk populations (individuals with a family history of Parkinson's and individuals over the age of fifty). The same micronutrient strategy can be used for secondary prevention in patients with early-stage Parkinson's who are not taking medication.

The current treatment of Parkinson's disease with medication and surgery is effective in improving the symptoms for a limited period of time, generally about five years. Treatment with L-dopa (levodopa) markedly improves symptoms, with the effectiveness of the drug lasting as long as DA neurons are alive. After this five-year window the toxic effects of L-dopa become the limiting factor for its continuation as effective therapy. None of the current medications or the surgical treatment affects the levels of oxidative stress and chronic inflammation; therefore, DA neurons continue to die despite standard therapy.

A clinical study using the above-referenced micronutrient strategy in combination with standard therapy should be initiated to improve the management and reduce Parkinson's progression. In the meantime, those individuals interested in utilizing the micronutrient approach to reduce the risk of the development and progression of Parkinson's disease, or those interested in improving the effectiveness of standard therapy in its management, might consider adopting these recommendations in consultation with their physician or health care professional.

6 Huntington's Disease

History, Incidence, Cost, and Causes

The wild-type (normal) Huntington gene plays an important role in the development of the human embryo and fetus. This gene is also considered essential for the survival of neurons in the brain, especially in the striatum and cortex. Huntington's disease is due to a mutation (change in gene structure) in the wild-type Huntington gene. The mutated form of the Huntington gene is referred to as Huntington's disease gene (HD).

Huntington's disease is a rare, fatal, familial neurodegenerative disease of the brain that exhibits a dominant mode of inheritance. This means that each child of a Huntington's disease parent has fifty-fifty odds of inheriting the HD gene. A child with the HD gene will develop the disease at an early age. The time of development of the symptoms of Huntington's may vary from one individual to another, but symptoms generally manifest when the individual is over thirty and under fifty. Juvenile Huntington's disease typically appears before the age of twenty and progresses rapidly. In adults the disease progresses over a period of ten to twenty-five years, until patients ultimately become unable to care for themselves. Muscle rigidity progresses at a rapid rate, leading to akinesia (loss of control of voluntary muscle movements). Huntington's disease is always fatal, and there is no cure for this disease. If a child has not inherited the HD gene, his or her subsequent children will not develop Huntington's disease.

In the brain, nerve cells in the striatum and cortex control movement, intellect, and emotion. These nerve cells are gradually destroyed in Huntington's, a disease that is also characterized by jerking, uncontrollable movements of the limbs, trunk, and face, a progressive loss of mental memory, and the development of psychiatric problems. There are no strategies to prevent or delay the onset of Huntington's. Existing treatment strategies focus on the management of its symptoms—with very limited success. The disease progresses despite treatment with medication, psychotherapy, physical therapy, and speech therapy.

This chapter briefly describes the history, incidence and prevalence, cost, and the symptoms and causes of Huntington's disease and provides scientific evidence in support of a hypothesis that increased oxidative stress, mitochondrial dysfunction, and chronic inflammation are the major biochemical defects that initiate its development and progression. These biochemical defects also damage neurotransmitter receptors and synaptic connections between nerve cells, which aggravate the symptoms of the disease.

HISTORY OF HUNTINGTON'S DISEASE

The symptoms of Huntington's disease (also known as Huntington's chorea) have been known for a long time. The word *chorea* is derived from the Latin. It originated from the Greek *khoria,* a choral dance. In the sixteenth century Paracelsus used the term *chorea* to describe movement disorders in humans, and a treatment for chorea was first proposed by Dr. Thomas Sydenham, a British physician (1624–1689). In 1872 a twenty-two-year-old American medical student by the name of George Huntington described the movement disorders in great detail and identified the disease as a hereditary disorder. This movement disorder now bears his name.

In 1993 fifty investigators from nine different countries identified a gene with several repeats of trinucleotide CAG (cytosine, adenine, and guanosine), which codes for the amino acid glutamine in Huntington's patients. In normal individuals CAG repeats are very few; however, CAG repeats are expanded severalfold in Huntington's disease. The HD gene is located on chromosome 4 (4p16.3) (MacDonald et al. 1993).

PREVALENCE, INCIDENCE, AND COST OF HUNTINGTON'S DISEASE

The prevalence of Huntington's disease appears to be highest in the USA, Europe, and Australia and lowest in Asia. It remains uncertain why Huntington's prevalence is so low in Asia compared to Western countries. Huntington's disease affects both males and females and all ethnic groups.

It is estimated that the incidence of Huntington's disease in the United States is approximately 1,550 cases per year.

TABLE 6.1. PREVALENCE OF HUNTINGTON'S DISEASE THROUGHOUT THE WORLD*

Country	Huntington's cases/ 100,000 individuals
United States, Europe, Australia	5.7
Asia	0.4
World	2.7

*From Pringsheim et al. 2012.

The annual costs of treating Huntington's disease may vary. The average annual medical cost per individual is about $10,500, but it could be as high as $47,000 if caregivers' costs are included.

SYMPTOMS OF HUNTINGTON'S DISEASE

In most cases the symptoms of Huntington's appear in young adult life and become progressively worse. As noted earlier, the major symptoms include movement disorders, cognitive dysfunction, and psychiatric problems. Movement disorders are characterized by uncontrolled movements (tics) in the fingers, feet, face, or trunk, which become more intense when the individuals are anxious or disturbed. As the disease progresses, other symptoms such as clumsiness, jaw clenching (bruxism), a loss of coordination and balance, slurred speech, swallowing/eating difficulties, uncontrolled continual muscular contractions (dystonia), and stumbling and falling may appear, as well as difficulty walking. Weight loss is a prominent feature of Huntington's disease.

The cognitive dysfunctions are characterized by a progressive loss of memory and an inability to concentrate, answer questions, and recognize familiar objects. Memory loss appears to develop later in the course of the disease.

The psychiatric problems attendant to Huntington's include depression, which appears early on. The major signs of depression include hostility/irritability, lack of energy, and an inability to experience pleasure in life. Some individuals may develop manic depression or bipolar disorder during the course of the disease. Others may exhibit psychotic behavior such as delusions, hallucinations, and/or unprovoked aggression and paranoia.

DEGENERATIVE CHANGES IN THE BRAIN

It has been reported that the Huntington's disease protein (HD protein) in the striatum and cortex is degraded into smaller fragments, which together with other proteins, form the insoluble aggregates that are toxic to nerve cells (Hoffner, Soues, and Djian 2007).

Aggregated HD protein fragments produce reactive oxygen

species (ROS), which contribute to the degeneration and death of nerve cells. In Huntington's patients degenerative changes in the nerve cells of the striatum appear early on and become severe as the disease progresses. Other regions of the brain such as the cortex, thalamus, and sub-thalamus also show degenerative changes with a progression of the disease. Within the striatum, the medium spiny projection neurons are selectively degenerated; however, interneurons are not significantly affected (Sadri-Vakili and Cha 2006).

CAUSES OF HUNTINGTON'S DISEASE

In Huntington's patients HD protein is found throughout the body, but it principally damages only the nerve cells in the brain. The exact reasons for this selective death of neurons by HD protein are unknown. I propose that the HD protein by itself may not be toxic to the nerve cells. However, when the HD protein is broken by the enzyme caspases (released from damaged mitochondria in the brain) into smaller fragments and form an aggregate with the help of copper or iron, it becomes toxic to the nerve cells. The aggregated form of HD protein causes damage to the nerve cells by generating free radicals. Damage to nerve cells is associated with the aberrant release and function of neurotransmitters such as dopamine, glutamate, and gamma-aminobutyric acid (GABA). In my view it is these biochemical defects in the brain that cause the death of nerve cells. The above-referenced biochemical defects do not occur in other organs outside the brain; therefore, the organs outside the brain are not affected by the HD protein.

Both chemically induced and genetically induced animal models of Huntington's disease and human Huntington's were used to investigate its mechanisms and to identify potential targets for the development of new drugs. The results of these studies showed that, as with Parkinson's disease, increased oxidative stress, mitochondrial dysfunction, and chronic inflammation play an important role in the disease's development and progression. The fact that increased oxidative stress occurs in individuals carrying the HD gene who are not displaying any symptoms suggests that increased oxidative stress is the key event that initiates the development of Huntington's disease and other biochemical defects. These other biochemical defects include the mitochondrial dysfunction, chronic inflammation, and glutamate release that occurs subsequent to increased oxidative stress. These biochemical abnormalities together with increased oxidative stress participate in the progression of the disease.

Increased chronic inflammation and reduced dopamine binding are also found in asymptomatic individuals; however, these changes may be caused by increased oxidative stress. The biochemical abnormalities referenced above are also found in symptomatic Huntington's patients, suggesting that these abnormalities also contribute to the progression of the disease (table 6.2). A simplified diagrammatic representation of the role of oxidative stress and the HD protein in the death of nerve cells is described in the box on page 118.

TABLE 6.2. INCREASED OXIDATIVE STRESS AND ITS CONSEQUENCES IN ASYMPTOMATIC HUNTINGTON'S PATIENTS COMPARED TO SYMPTOMATIC HUNTINGTON'S PATIENTS AND NORMAL HEALTHY INDIVIDUALS*

Type of patients	Increased oxidative stress	Increased inflammation	Increased GABA	Increased dopamine binding
Asymptomatic	Yes	Yes	Yes	Yes
Symptomatic	Yes	Yes	Yes	Yes
Normal	No	No	No	No

*Legend:

Asymptomatic: an individual carrying the HD gene but displaying no symptoms of the disease

Symptomatic: an individual displaying symptoms of Huntington's disease

GABA: gamma-aminobutyric acid

Diagrammatic Representations of Various Pathways Affected by Increased Oxidative Stress, Which Cause Degeneration and Death of Neurons in Huntington's Disease

Increased oxidative stress→→Mitochondrial dysfunction→→Releases caspases→→Cleaves HD protein into smaller fragments→→Forms aggregate with copper or iron→→Produces free radicals→→Damage to nerve cells→→Release of glutamate→→Death of nerve cells

Increased oxidative stress→→Mitochondrial dysfunction→→Decrease of PGC-1alpha→→Increase of free radicals→→Death of nerve cells

Increased oxidative stress→→Damage to DNA→→Activate IKKB→→Release of caspases→→Cleaves HD protein into smaller fragments→→Forms aggregate with copper or iron→→Produces free radicals→→Damage to nerve cells→→Release of glutamate→→Death of nerve cells

Aggregation of HD protein fragments→→Increase of free radicals→→Damage to nerve cells→→Increase of chronic inflammation→→Release of pro-inflammatory cytokines and free radicals→→Death of nerve cells

Aggregation of HD protein fragments→→Migrate to the nucleus→→Deacetylation of histone→→Suppressed gene expression→→Degeneration of nerve cells→→Death of nerve cells

EVIDENCE OF INCREASED OXIDATIVE STRESS IN HUNTINGTON'S DISEASE

Studies of Chemically Induced Animal Models of Huntington's Disease

Administration of quinolinic acid, an NMDA (N-methyl-D-aspartate) receptor agonist, or 3-nitropropionic acid (3-NP), an inhibitor of mitochondrial dehydrogenase activity, directly into the striatum region of the rat brain produced some biochemical, morphological, and behavioral characteristics of human Huntington's. It has been reported that NADPH (nicotinamide adenine dinucleotide pohosphate) oxidase activity, which produces superoxide anions, increased in the quinolinic-acid-treated neurons in the striatum. Treatment with Apocynin, a specific inhibitor of NADPH oxidase, decreased quinolinic acid–induced NADPH oxidase activity, lipid peroxidation, circling behavior, and degenerative changes in the brain (Maldonado et al. 2010).

Increased oxidative and nitrosylative stress contribute to the degeneration of nerve cells caused by treatment with quinolinic acid (Perez-De La Cruz et al. 2005) or 3-NP (Tunez and Santamaria 2009).

The results of studies of chemically induced animal Huntington's models support the hypothesis that increased oxidative stress is one of the earliest biochemical defects that initiates development and progression.

Studies of Genetically Induced Animal Models

Some genetic mouse and rat models of Huntington's—in which the HD gene has been inserted—are available to investigate the biochemical defects and defects in the regulation of genes that are found in Huntington's. These animal models mimic the degenerative changes in the striatum and cortex regions of the brain and also mimic symptoms that are observed in the human disease. Transgenic Huntington's mouse models with smaller fragments of the HD gene (R6/1 and R6/2 mice) or with a full-length HD gene (YAC128 mice) exhibited rapid changes in gene expressions in the neurons of the striatum similar to those observed in human Huntington's (Kuhn et al. 2007).

It is known that caspases enzymes are released when mitochondria are damaged. It was demonstrated that the expression of caspase-1 and caspase-3 genes, as well as the activities of caspase-1 and caspase-2 enzymes, were enhanced in a transgenic Huntington's mouse model (Sanchez Mejia and Friedlander 2001). This is consistent with the observation that increased activity of caspase-1 enzyme is present in the autopsied brain samples of Huntington's patients. The increased activities of caspases cause cleavage of the HD proteins into smaller fragments, which aggregate and then cause the death of nerve cells via increased oxidative stress. The degree of enhancement (of the activities of the caspases) correlated with the progression of the disease in these mice. Inhibitors of activities of caspases delayed the onset of symptoms in the transgenic mouse model. The results of the genetic animal models suggest that caspase-induced cleavage of the HD protein is necessary for the degeneration of the nerve cells in the brain.

Studies in Humans

There is substantial evidence for the involvement of increased oxidative stress in the development and progression of Huntington's disease (Browne and Beal 2006). Metabolic defects in the brain and muscle, and progressive weight loss, have been observed in Huntington's patients. In addition, mitochondrial dysfunction due to reduced activities of the respiratory chain complexes have been found in the autopsied brain samples.

It has been suggested that HD proteins accumulate in mitochondria and cause mitochondrial dysfunction, which is associated with the progression of the disease (Browne 2008). It's possible that HD proteins bind with the respiratory chain complexes and reduce their activities, resulting in the reduced energy production that is one of the disease's characteristic features. Mitochondrial dysfunction can increase the production of reactive oxygen species (ROS).

In a clinical study of 19 Huntington's patients and 47 age-sex-matched healthy individuals, a 20 percent increase in plasma lipid peroxidation levels and a 28 percent decrease in glutathione levels were found in Huntington's patients compared to those of healthy individuals. Similar changes in the levels of these markers of oxidative stress were observed in 11 asymptomatic HD gene carriers compared to those in 22 age-sex-matched healthy individuals who did not carry the HD gene.

These results suggest that increased oxidative stress occurs prior to the onset of Huntington's symptoms in asymptomatic individuals carrying the HD gene (Hickey et al. 2008). Increased oxidative stress and mitochondrial dysfunction as evidenced by decreased activities of complexes II, III, and IV in the striatum have been consistently observed in Huntington's patients. The increased oxidative stress in individuals carrying the HD gene with no symptoms of the disease provides the strongest support for the hypothesis that increased oxidative stress initiates degenerative changes in the nerve cells.

In another clinical study, 16 Huntington's patients and 36 age-sex-matched healthy individuals were recruited to evaluate the role of oxidative stress in disease progression. The results showed that markers of oxidative stress—such as the levels of 8-hydroxydeoxyguanosine (8-OHdG) in the leukocytes and malondialdehyde (MDA) in the plasma—were increased. The activities of antioxidant enzymes—such as erythrocyte Cu/Zn superoxide dismutase (Cu/Zn-SOD) and glutathione peroxidase—were reduced in Huntington's patients compared to those in healthy individuals (Chen et al. 2007). It is interesting to note that plasma MDA levels were significantly correlated with the severity of the disease.

Increased mitochondrial DNA defects that were possibly induced by increased oxidative stress and/or by HD protein were also observed in the autopsied brain samples of Huntington's patients compared to those of healthy individuals.

These results suggest that increased oxidative stress and mitochondrial dysfunction play an important role in disease progression.

Analysis of the autopsied brain tissues from Huntington's patients revealed that activities of oxidative phosphorylation enzymes were reduced only in the basal ganglia (Browne et al. 1997). In addition, the levels of markers of oxidative stress increased in the caudate of the diseased brain. These results suggest that increased oxidative stress and energy insufficiency contribute to the progression of Huntington's disease.

Aggregation of HD Protein

Enzyme caspases released from the damaged mitochondria break HD protein into smaller fragments and fragmented HD protein aggregates. The aggregated form of HD protein causes the selective death of nerve cells in the striatum and cortex. These changes were also observed in the autopsied brain samples of patients with Huntington's disease, as well as in a Huntington's mouse model expressing a full-length HD gene (YAC72 mice) (Hermel et al. 2004).

Trace metals such as copper and iron are essential for survival; however, increased levels of these trace metals can cause aggregation of HD protein fragments. In addition, increased oxidative stress can also cause aggregation of HD protein (Goswami et al. 2006).

Aggregated forms of HD protein induce degeneration and death of the nerve cells by producing excessive amounts of free radicals (Rivera-Mancia et al. 2010; Hands et al. 2011).

It has been reported that interactions between copper and HD protein caused increased oxidative stress by forming aggregates that contribute to the degeneration of nerve cells in Huntington's disease (Fox et al. 2007). The aggregated form of HD protein fragments bind with mitochondria to induce mitochondrial dysfunction. In addition, aggregated HD protein migrates to the nucleus where it can impair the expression of genes. These data suggest that increased oxidative stress and energy insufficiency due to mitochondrial dysfunction contribute to the progression of the disease.

Cell-Culture Studies

Increased oxidative stress also inhibited proteasome activity in cultured nerve cells (that were growing in petri dishes) expressing the HD gene. The inhibition of proteasome activity may result in the accumulation of faulty proteins within the nerve cells, which can cause degeneration (Goswami et al. 2006). Furthermore, an overexpression of the antioxidant enzyme superoxide dismutase-1 (SOD-1) reversed oxidative stress-induced proteasome inhibition and HD protein aggregation and death in those cultured nerve cells expressing the HD gene. These studies suggest that increased oxidative stress plays a central role in development and progression. Increased oxidative stress also activates microglia, which releases free radicals and pro-inflammatory cytokines that are very toxic to the nerve cells.

EVIDENCE FOR INCREASED CHRONIC INFLAMMATION IN HUNTINGTON'S DISEASE

An examination of autopsied human brain samples revealed that activated microglia is present in the area of neuronal loss. Measurements of a radioactive marker of microglia activation, ^{11}C (R)-PK11195, and a radioactive marker of the dopamine D2 receptor ^{11}C raclopride by PET (positron emission tomography) in Huntington's patients at different stages of the disease revealed that an increase in microglia activation correlated with the severity of the disease. In addition, a reduction in the binding of dopamine D2 receptors and in the Unified Huntington Disease Scale Score were also decreased in these patients (Pavese et al. 2006).

Using the same radioactive markers by PET technique it was demonstrated that microglia activation was also observed in individuals who were carrying the HD gene but not displaying any symptoms. This result suggested that microglia activation, a marker of chronic inflammation, participates in the initiation of damage to the nerve cells and that it was associated with the subclinical progression (Tai et al. 2007). Furthermore, degeneration of the sensorimotor striatum, substantia nigra, orbitofrontal, and anterior prefrontal cortex regions of the brain also occurred in asymptomatic patients. In addition, the binding of dopamine D2/D3 receptors was reduced, and the activation of microglia was increased in asymptomatic patients.

The above defects progressively increased in the striatum and cortex of symptomatic patients. From these results it was concluded that activated microglia exist in the areas of the brain that are responsible for cognitive function (Politis et al. 2011).

Using nerve cells from the cortex area of the brain, which were engineered to express HD protein, it was demonstrated that the number of activated microglia increased. In addition, the levels of interleukin-6 (IL-6) and complement protein 1q (markers of chronic inflammation) increased (Kraft et al. 2012).

A clinical study reported that plasma levels of IL-6, a marker of pro-inflammatory cytokine, were elevated in asymptomatic individuals carrying the HD gene 16 years before the onset of symptoms of the disease (Bjorkqvist et al. 2008). In addition, monocytes from the asymptomatic Huntington's patients were hyperactive. These monocytes can release excessive amounts of free radicals and pro-inflammatory cytokines that are toxic to nerve cells. These results suggest that activated microglia cause degeneration of nerve cells by releasing toxic products such as free radicals, pro-inflammatory cytokines, complement proteins, and prostaglandins. The presence of products of chronic inflammation in the asymptomatic patients suggests that chronic inflammation plays a role in the development of this disease.

Blood levels of pro-inflammatory cytokine IL-23 and the soluble human leukocyte antigen-G (sHLA-G) were increased in most of the presenting, severe cases, and a significant correlation between IL-23 and the severity of the disease was observed (Forrest et al. 2010). These results suggest that pro-inflammatory cytokines participate in Huntington's progression.

The IkB kinase B (IKKB) is a regulator of inflammation in the brain. Pro-inflammatory cytokines accumulate in the serum and brain of asymptomatic and symptomatic patients, and the levels of pro-inflammatory cytokines correlate with disease progression. Oxidative stress-induced damage to DNA activates IKKB. This triggers the release of enzyme caspases, which break the HD protein into smaller fragments that accumulate in the brain and are toxic in the aggregated form (Khoshnan and Patterson 2011).

The role of chronic inflammation in the development and progression of Huntington's is further supported by observations in which treatment with nonsteroidal anti-inflammatory agents produced beneficial effects in animal models.

Treatment of a Huntington's rat model (quinolinic acid–induced Huntington's) with celecoxib, a selective inhibitor of cyclooxygenase-2 (COX-2), markedly improved behavior and biochemical changes in the brains of Huntington's rats, suggesting that activation of immune cells like microglia may contribute to disease development (Kalonia and Kumar 2011).

Treatment of Huntington's rats with verapamil or diltiazem (FDA-approved drugs for other conditions in humans) for twenty-one days improved motor function and reduced oxidative damage and markers of pro-inflammatory cytokines (TNF-alpha, IL-6, and caspase-3) (Kalonia, Kumar, and Kumar 2011). The significance of these results in the treatment of Huntington's in humans remains uncertain.

DEFECTS IN MITOCHONDRIAL FUNCTIONS IN HUNTINGTON'S DISEASE

Most free radicals are produced in the mitochondria, which are easily damaged by free radicals. Damaged mitochondria release more free radicals and enzyme caspases, all of which are toxic to the nerve cells. Mitochondrial dysfunction is associated with certain neurodegenerative diseases including Huntington's. Increased oxidative stress is one of the factors that can induce mitochondrial dysfunction. In addition, aggregated forms of HD protein also induce mitochondrial dysfunction by inhibiting activities of respiratory complexes (playing a role in producing energy) and reducing mitochondrial DNA activity.

In Huntington's patients the number of mitochondria in the spiny neurons of the striatum decreased. Furthermore, the peroxisome proliferator-activated gamma receptor-coactivator gamma-1alpha (PGC-1 alpha), a key regulator of the gene responsible for energy production and for the formation of new mitochondria, was reduced with increased severity of Huntington's disease. These results suggest that mitochondrial dysfunction plays an important role in disease development (Kim et al. 2010).

Mitochondrial dysfunction produces reduced energy and releases enzyme caspases (responsible for cleaving HD protein into smaller fragments) and excessive amounts of free radicals. The results suggest that overexpression of PGC-1 alpha may prevent mitochondrial dysfunction and reduce neurodegeneration. Indeed, overexpression of PGC-1 alpha partially reversed the toxic effect of HD protein in the nerve cells obtained from the striatum.

In addition, administration of PGC-1 alpha directly into the striatum reduced degeneration of nerve cells in transgenic Huntington's mice (Cui et al. 2006).

Using the mouse model it was shown that elevation of the PGC-1 alpha level eliminated HD protein aggregation and prevented neurodegeneration by reducing oxidative stress (Tsunemi et al. 2012). It was further demonstrated that PGC-1 alpha promoted turnover of HD protein and eliminated protein aggregates. Therefore, it was suggested that PGC-1 alpha could be used as a target for developing new therapeutic agents. Thus, mitochondrial dysfunction enhances disease progression. It appears that an administration of PGC-1 alpha or elevation of PGC-1 alpha protects the nerve cells against the toxic effects of the aggregated form of HD protein fragments by reducing oxidative stress in animal models.

DEREGULATION OF GENE EXPRESSION IN HUNTINGTON'S DISEASE

It has been demonstrated that mitogen- and stress-activated kinase (MSK-1), a nuclear protein kinase, was reduced in the autopsied samples of the striatum of Huntington's patients as well as in the striatum of animal models (Martin et al. 2011). Restoring MSK-1 expression in neurons from the striatum prevented HD protein–induced degeneration and death of the nerve cells. Furthermore, deletion of MSK-1 in normal mice showed spontaneous degeneration of nerve cells in the striatum as they aged and increased sensitivity of nerve cells to mitochondrial neurotoxin 3-NP.

HISTONE DEACETYLATION IN HUNTINGTON'S DISEASE

Acetylation and deacetylation of histone protein regulate gene expression. Acetylation of histone increases the rate of gene expression, whereas deacetylation of histone suppresses gene expression. Defects in the regulation of gene expression have been implicated in Huntington's development and progression. In animal models HD protein causes deacetylation of histone. Deacetylation of histone inhibits the rate of gene expression that causes degeneration of nerve cells in the brain.

Inhibitors of histone deacetylase (HDAC) produce some beneficial effects in several animal models (Sadri-Vakili and Cha 2006); however, their therapeutic value is limited by their toxicity. Chronic oral administration of an HDAC inhibitor, HDACi 4b, beginning and after the onset of motor deficits, significantly improved motor performance, overall appearance, and body weight in the transgenic mouse model of Huntington's. These changes were associated with improvement in brain size and reduction in degeneration of nerve cells in the striatum.

In addition, treatment with HDACi 4b prevented an HD protein–induced reduction in alterations in gene expression (Thomas et al. 2008). The effectiveness of HDAC inhibitor HDACi 4b has not been evaluated in human disease.

REDUCTION IN PALMITOYLATION OF PROTEIN IN HUNTINGTON'S DISEASE

Changes in the structure of proteins by the lipid palmitate are important for the appropriate functioning of Huntington protein. The process of changing the structure of protein by the lipid palmitate is called "palmitoylation." Palmitoylation of proteins is regulated by two functionally opposing enzyme palmitoyl acyltransferases (PATs), which add palmitate to the proteins, and acyl protein thioesterases, which remove palmitate from the proteins. This process is particularly important for the development and proper functioning of synapses in the brain.

It has been reported that the wild-type Huntington protein is palmitoylated by Huntington-interacting protein-14 (HIP-14) (Yanai et al. 2006). In Huntington's disease the interaction between HD protein and HIP-14 is reduced, causing a decrease in the palmitoylation of HD protein. Reduced palmitoylation of the HD protein increases the rate of protein aggregation and degeneration of nerve cells in the striatum. On the other hand, overexpression of HIP-14 can increase the palmitoylation of the HD protein that markedly reduces aggregation of the HD protein fragments. This study suggests that increased levels of HIP-14 may prevent development and progression.

The protective role of HIP-14 was further confirmed by a study in which deletion of HIP-14 induced degenerative changes in the neurons of the striatum and behavior deficits in mice similar to those found in the human disease (Young et al. 2012).

IMPAIRED NEUROTRANSMITTER RECEPTORS
IN HUNTINGTON'S DISEASE

Extensive studies using primarily the cell-culture Huntington's model, chemically induced rodent models, or transgenic rodent models revealed that the release and transmission of various neurotransmitters such as glutamate, GABA, dopamine, and cannabinoid, are impaired. Impaired release of neurotransmitters and their respective defective receptors contributes to development and progression. The exact mechanisms are not known.

Increased levels of glutamate in the extracellular fluid of the striatum contribute to the degeneration and death of nerve cells. The toxic effect of glutamate is mediated through NMDA receptors. Treatment of striatal precursor cell line expressing full-length wild-type Huntington gene or HD gene with an N-methy-D-aspartate (NMDA) agonist caused early death in nerve cells expressing the HD gene compared to those nerve cells expressing the wild-type Huntington gene (Xifro et al. 2008). The nerve cells expressing the HD gene had higher levels of calcineurin A, a calcium-dependent phosphatase-3. The activity of calcineurin A was further increased after treatment of nerve cells expressing the HD gene with an NMDA receptor agonist. This suggested that higher levels of calcineurin A in nerve cells expressing the HD gene may account for the early death of nerve cells in the striatum. Indeed, treatment with a calcineurin inhibitor FK-506 reduced death more in the nerve cells expressing the HD gene than in the nerve cells expressing the wild-type Huntington gene. These results suggest that high levels of calcineurin A in the nerve cells expressing the HD gene may increase their sensitivity to glutamate.

Evidence for the role of glutamate in the development of Huntington's was evidenced by the early presence of increased levels of quinolinate, an NMDA receptor agonist, in patients with the disease. Using a transgenic mouse model (YAC128) it was demonstrated that the nerve cells in the striatum exhibited enhanced sensitivity to NMDA receptor agonists before the onset of HD-associated changes in the brain. However, after the onset of HD-associated changes, nerve cells in the striatum showed resistance to quinolinate (Graham et al. 2009). These paradoxical results cannot be explained at this time, given that the NMDA receptor agonist contributes to the degeneration of nerve cells irrespective of the stage of the disease.

Another study reported that stimulation of the N-methyl-D-aspartate (NMDA) receptor by glutamate contributes to the degeneration and death of the nerve cells. This is substantiated by observations that showed that administration of NMDA receptor agonists into the striatum of rodents or nonhuman primates induced degenerative changes in the nerve cells, which is characteristic of Huntington's disease (Fan and Raymond 2007).

Reduced Glutamate Transporter Proteins

The two major glutamate transporter proteins, glutamate transporter-1 (GLT-1) and glutamate-aspartate transporter (GLAST), are primarily located in the astrocytes of the adult brain. These transporter proteins play an important role in maintaining normal levels of glutamate in the striatum. In the transgenic mouse model (R6/2 mice) release of vitamin C from the striatum into the extracellular fluid is reduced, together with the reduction in a GLT-1-dependent uptake of glutamate. These changes reduce the levels of vitamin C and increase the levels of glutamate in the extracellular (outside the nerve cells in the brain) fluid of the striatal neurons. Reduced antioxidant levels and increased glutamate levels contribute to the degeneration of nerve cells in the striatum (Miller et al. 2012).

It has been reported that injection of vitamin C restored the extracellular levels of vitamin C in transgenic Huntington's mice (R6/2 mice) to the levels in wild-type mice and reversed and normalized the function of nerve cells in the striatum of Huntington's disease (Rebec, Conroy, and Barton 2006).

GABA Receptors

In the transgenic mouse model it was found that GABA (A) receptor-mediated inhibitory transmission is reduced, probably due to a loss of GABA receptors (Yuen et al. 2012). The reduced inhibitory synaptic transmission may lead to increased excitatory activity due to enhanced levels of glutamate, which contributes to the death of nerve cells.

Dopamine Receptors

It appears that dopamine neurons in the striatum primarily degenerate in Huntington's patients. Using neuroblastoma (NB) cells with the dopamine D1 receptor expressing wild-type Huntington protein or HD protein, it was demonstrated that HD protein aggregates were present in the nucleus and the cytoplasm of NB cells expressing the HD gene. Low doses of selective dopamine D1 receptor agonists increased the aggregation of HD proteins in the nucleus but decreased the number of aggregates in the cytoplasm (Robinson, Lebel, and Cyr 2008). Aggregated HD protein fragments in the nucleus may reduce gene expressions that contribute to the degeneration of nerve cells in the brain.

Using normal neurons obtained from the striatum-expressing HD gene, it was demonstrated that low doses of dopamine act synergistically with the HD gene in activating the transcriptional factor c-JUN and in increasing the number of HD protein aggregates in both the nucleus and the cytoplasm (Charvin et al. 2005). Furthermore, the effects of dopamine on HD protein aggregates and c-JUN were reversed by vitamin C or by SP-600125, a selective inhibitor of c-JUN. This would suggest that dopamine-induced degenerative changes in the neurons of the striatum-expressing HD gene are due to an excessive production of free radicals.

Like the dopamine D1 receptor agonist, the dopamine D2 receptor agonist also caused HD protein aggregations, which were blocked by a dopamine D2 receptor antagonist. The combination of vitamin C and dopamine D2 receptor antagonist was more effective in reducing the formation of HD protein aggregates and death of nerve cells in the striatum than the individual agents. Using rats expressing the HD gene, it was observed that chronic treatment with haloperidol, an antagonist of dopamine D2 receptor, protected neurons in the striatum from degeneration and death, suggesting that the activation of dopamine D2 receptors contribute to HD protein aggregation and neurodegeneration (Charvin et al. 2008).

Impairments of dopamine release and uptake progressed as a function of age in the transgenic mouse model of Huntington's (R6/1) (Ortiz et al. 2011). Dopamine release was also reduced in a transgenic rat model, and this contributed to motor deficiency as evidenced by gait disturbances in these animals (Ortiz et al. 2012).

It should be noted that the defects in dopamine neuron function have been observed in both symptomatic and asymptomatic patients. Using a radioactive marker of specific agonist of dopamine D2 receptors 11C-raclopride, the binding of dopamine D2 receptors in 16 symptomatic and 11 asymptomatic patients was determined by positron emission tomography (PET) technology. The results showed that the binding of dopamine D2 receptors was reduced in most symptomatic and asymptomatic patients. This study suggests that a reduced binding of dopamine D2 receptors occurs in individuals carrying the HD gene without any symptoms. Symptomatic patients showed increased deficits in attention and executive functions (Pavese et al. 2010).

The severity of clinical symptoms of the disease, such as chorea and cognitive test performance, were correlated with the degree of reduction in the binding of dopamine D2 receptors (Esmaeilzadeh et al. 2011). These results suggest that reduced binding of dopamine D2 receptors should also be considered as an early event that participates in disease development.

Adenosine Receptors

It has been reported that treatment with an adenosine A (2A) receptor (A2ARs) agonist improved some of the symptoms of Huntington's in a mouse model (R6/2 mice) (Martire et al. 2007). This study suggests that activation of A2ARs may have protective value (at least in the mouse model). If this is the case, then the deletion of A2ARs should enhance the symptoms. Indeed, genetic deletion of A2ARs aggravated the motor performance and reduced the survival of the transgenic mouse model (N171-82Q mice) (Mievis, Blum, and Ledent 2011).

Brain-Derived Growth Factor (BDNF)

Brain-derived neurotrophic factor (BDNF) is essential for the survival of brain neurons. In addition, this neurotrophic factor is needed for the correct synaptic activity of neurons in the cortex and striatum regions of the brain, as well as the survival of GABAergic medium-size spiny neurons in the striatum that are lost in Huntington's disease. Indeed, examination of autopsied samples of the diseased brain showed a major loss of BDNF protein in the striatum. Thus, a loss of BDNF may contribute to the degeneration of neurons in the striatum associated with Huntington's (Zuccato and Cattaneo 2007).

Cannabinoid Receptors

Cannabinoids are chemical compounds primarily found in cannabis plants. These compounds activate cannabinoid receptors (CBs). Cannabinoid receptors in the adult human brain are primarily located in the forebrain, midbrain, and in the brain's hind areas that regulate cognitive function, movement, and the motor and sensory functions of the autonomic nervous system (Glass, Dragunow, and Faull 1997). The levels of CB1 and CB2 receptors were reduced in the striatum and cortex of the diseased brain.

CB1 Receptors

Loss of CB1 receptors was observed at the early stage of Huntington's in the autopsied brain samples of Huntington's patients (Glass, Dragunow, and Faull 2000).

This was confirmed by the PET technology in which a radioactive novel CB1 ligand N-[2-(3-cyano-phenyl)-3-(4-(2-^{18}F-fluorethoxy) phenyl)-1-methylpropyl]-2-(5-methyl-2-pyridyloxyl)-2-methylpropon-amide was administered in 20 symptomatic patients and 14 healthy individuals. The results showed that the levels of CB1 receptors decreased throughout the gray matter of the cerebellum and brain stem in the early stage of disease more than in healthy individuals (Van Laere et al. 2010). This study suggested that enhanced levels of CB1 receptors may be of protective value.

Indeed, it was observed that increased levels of CB1 receptors reduced the rate of progression of the disease in the Huntington's transgenic mouse model (R6/1 mice) (Glass et al. 2004).

Deletion of CB1 receptors aggravated the symptoms and caused neurodegeneration and molecular defects in transgenic mice (Blazquez et al. 2011). Furthermore, administration of the endogenous cannabinoid receptor agonist (delta-9-tetrahydrocannabinol) prevented the effect of deletion of CB1 receptors in these transgenic mice.

These data suggest that agonists of CB1 receptors may be useful in improving symptoms. Indeed, administration of the CB1 agonist (WIN 55, 212-2) prevented the development of degenerative changes in the brains in a rat model. This effect of the CB1 receptor agonist was prevented by the CB1 receptor antagonist (AM251) (Pintor et al. 2006).

CB2 Receptors

It was demonstrated that CB2 receptors are present in small amounts in the striatum, but they are abundantly located in microglia and astrocytes, suggesting that protective effects of the agonist of CB2 receptors are mediated by astrocytes and microglia (Sagredo et al. 2009).

Activation of the cannabinoid receptor CB2 reduced activation of microglia. This is shown by the fact that deletion of CB2 receptors in the mouse model accelerated the onset of motor deficits and increased their severity. Treatment of mice with a CB2 receptor agonist extended life span and suppressed motor deficits, synapse loss, and brain inflammation, whereas a CB2 receptor antagonist blocked these effects (Bouchard et al. 2012). Furthermore, treatment with a CB2 receptor agonist reduced blood levels of IL-6, which was elevated in Huntington's mice. Treatment with an antibody, against IL-6, also improved motor function in these mice.

CONCLUDING REMARKS

Huntington's disease that is caused by a mutation in the wild-type Huntington gene is a rare, fatal, familial disease of the brain in which neurons (primarily found in the striatum and cortex) that regulate movement, intellect, and emotion are gradually destroyed. The mutated Huntington gene is referred to as the HD gene. The HD gene has repeated expansion of trinucleotide CAG (cytosine, adenine, and guanosine) that codes for glutamine much more than the wild-type Huntington gene does. Huntington's disease is characterized by jerking, uncontrollable movements of the limbs, trunk, and face (collectively known as chorea); progressive loss of mental abilities; and the development of psychiatric problems. The offspring of a Huntington's parent have a fifty-fifty chance of inheriting the HD gene.

There is no cure for this disease, and there are no strategies for preventing or delaying its onset. Current treatment with medication, psychotherapy, physical therapy, and speech therapy is unsatisfactory. It appears that increased oxidative stress, chronic inflammation, and release of glutamate are early events in the disease's development, and these biological processes also participate in its progression. Abnormalities in neurotransmitter receptors such as glutamate, gamma-aminobutyric acid (GABA), dopamine, adenosine, and cannabinoid, appear as the disease progresses and enhance its rate of progression. Other molecular defects, such as defects in gene expressions at the nuclear and mitochondrial levels, may occur at the disease's early stage and progress from there.

7 Prevention and Management of Huntington's Disease with Vitamins and Antioxidants

At the present time there are no preventive strategies to delay the onset of the symptoms of Huntington's disease in humans, nor is there a cure for it. The primary aim of the current treatment strategy is to manage the symptoms of the disease. Despite treatment, the disease progresses and patients die. As we have stated earlier, current therapies include medication, psychotherapy, speech therapy, and physical therapy, which are of minimal value. In addition, drugs used for the treatment of Huntington's have serious, deleterious side effects.

Growing evidence from human and animal models has established that increased oxidative stress and chronic inflammation play an important role in the development and progression of Huntington's disease. Even asymptomatic individuals carrying the HD gene without any symptoms show the presence of increased oxidative stress and chronic inflammation in the brain as well as in the plasma. Thus, reducing oxidative stress and chronic inflammation appears to be one way of preventing and/or delaying the onset of Huntington's symptoms in humans.

The same strategy in combination with standard therapy may improve the management of this disease. An optimal reduction in the levels of oxidative stress and chronic inflammation would require an elevation of antioxidant enzymes as well as dietary and endogenous antioxidants. The use of one or two antioxidants is unlikely to achieve this goal. Unfortunately, most previous studies of Huntington's disease have utilized a single antioxidant such as B vitamins, vitamin C, vitamin E, n-acetylcysteine, alpha-lipoic acid, coenzyme Q10, L-carnitine, lycopene, curcumin, resveratrol, *Ginkgo biloba,* epigallocatechin, or melatonin. These agents have produced some beneficial effects primarily in animal models.

Medication used in standard therapy does not affect oxidative stress or chronic inflammation, and therefore neurons continue to die despite drug treatment. Additional approaches should be developed to prevent the loss of the brain's neurons, which would reduce the progression of the disease and be more effective in improving the symptoms.

This chapter briefly describes studies of individual antioxidants in animal models and human Huntington's disease. It also presents scientific rationale for the use of a preparation of micronutrients for the prevention and/or delayed onset of the symptoms and, in combination with standard therapy, for the improved management.

STUDIES OF VITAMINS, ANTIOXIDANTS, AND PHENOLIC COMPOUNDS ON THE PREVENTION AND PROGRESSION OF HUNTINGTON'S DISEASE

Alpha-Tocopherol (Vitamin E) Study in Humans

In a clinical study of 73 patients with Huntington's it was found that treatment with d-alpha-tocopherol (natural vitamin E) had no effect on neurological symptoms or psychiatric problems; however, some beneficial effects on neurological symptoms were observed during the early course of the disease (Peyser et al. 1995) when these substances were administered. These results suggest that antioxidants may be of some value in delaying the onset of the symptoms of the disease.

Study of an Animal Model with Vitamin C

Using a transgenic mouse model (R6/2 mice), it was shown that administration of vitamin C at the beginning of the onset of symptoms restored a release of vitamin C in the striatum to normal level and improved motor performance without altering overall motor activity (Rebec et al. 2003).

Studies of an Animal Model with N-acetylcysteine (NAC)

Given that mitochondrial dysfunction is present in Huntington's, the efficacy of n-acetylcysteine in improving mitochondrial function in a 3-nitropropionic acid (3-NP)–induced rat model was tested (Sandhir et al. 2012). The results showed that rats treated with 3-NP exhibited inhibition of the activities of the brain's mitochondrial complexes II, IV, and V in the striatum, similar to those found in the human disease.

In addition, an increased production of reactive oxygen species (ROS) and lipid peroxidation were observed in the brain mitochondria of 3-NP treated rats. Increased levels of cytochrome c in the cytoplasm, mitochondrial swelling, and increased expression of caspase-3 and p53 were found in the brains of NP-3 treated animals. Damage to the brain included degneration of neurons and gliosis (increased prolifration of glia cells), and behavioral changes included motor functional deficits and cognitive dysfunction. Treatment of Huntington's animals with NAC reversed 3-NP-induced mitochondrial dysfunction and deficits in motor and cognitive function. This study suggests that the effect of 3-NP induced degenerative changes in neurons and behavioral deficits are due to an increased production of free radicals.

Study of an Animal Model with Alpha-Lipoic Acid

Treatment of transgenic Huntington's mice with alpha-lipoic acid, an endogenous antioxidant, increased the survival of transgenic mice (Andreassen et al. 2001). This study suggests that increased oxidative stress contributes to the degeneraion of nerve cells in the brains of transgenic Huntington's mice.

Studies of an Animal Model with Coenzyme Q10

Using a transgenic mouse model, it was demonstrated that mice fed with 0.2 and 0.6 percent of coenzyme Q10 in their diet improved early behavioral deficits and normalized some defects in gene expression without altering the levels of HD protein aggregates in the striatum (Hickey et al. 2012). It was noted that coenzyme Q10 at a low dose was more effective than that observed at a high dose. Treatment of wild-type mice with low-dose coenzyme Q10 (0.2 percent) induced motor deficits. This deleterious effect of coenzyme Q10 may be unique to mice, given that no harmful effects of high doses of coenzyme Q10 have been observed in humans.

In another study using the transgenic mouse model (R6/2 mice) it was demonstrated that brain levels of coenzyme Q9 and coenzyme Q10 were lower in transgenic Huntington's mice than in wild-type mice. Oral administration of coenzyme Q10 increased the plasma levels of coenzyme Q10 and the brain levels of coenzyme Q9 and coenzyme Q10 in transgenic Huntington's mice. Treatment with high doses of coenzyme Q10 significantly extended the survival of transgenic mice in a dose-dependent manner and improved motor function. It reduced weight loss and HD protein aggregation and stemmed the loss of neurons (Smith et al. 2006).

A combination of coenzyme Q10 and creatine produced an added protective effect in improving motor performance and extending the survival of transgenic Huntington's mice (Yang et al. 2009). Thus, treatment with coenzyme Q10 produces some beneficial effects in improving the survival and motor functions of transgenic mice.

Studies of an Animal Model with L-Carnitine

Using 3-NP and quinoliic acid–induced Huntington's rat models, it was demonstrated that treatment with L-carnitine prevented 3-NP-induced motor deficits (Silva-Adaya et al. 2008).

L-carnitine treatment also reduced quinolinic acid–induced gliosis and 3-NP-induced brain damage in the Huntington's rat.

Administration of L-carnitine increased survival, improved motor function, and reduced neuronal loss and the number of intranuclear HD protein aggregates. It was proposed that L-carnitine protected neurons by reducing oxidative damage (Vamos et al. 2010).

Study of an Animal Model with Lycopene and Epigallocatechin

Treatment of a Huntington's rat model with lycopene and epigallocatechin improved memory function and restored glutathione levels and glutathione-S-transferase activity in the striatum, hippocampus, and cortex areas. Furthermore, pretreatment with arginine (which produces nitric oxide), increased the effectiveness of lycopene and epigallocatechin in protecting nerve cells from 3-NP-induced damage (Kumar and Kumar 2009).

Study of an Animal Model with Melatonin

The hormone melatonin is secreted by the pineal gland and is necessary for sleep. Melatonin also exhibits antioxidant activity. A study has reported that supplementation with melatonin delayed the onset of Huntington's and its associated mortality in a transgenic mouse model (Wang et al. 2011). A loss of type 1 melatonin receptors (MT1) has been found in human Huntington's as well as in the transgenic mouse model. It has been reported that high levels of MT1 receptors are present in the mitochondria of the brains of wild-type mice; however, in the transgenic mouse HD model, reduced levels of MT1 receptors were found (Wang et al. 2011). Treatment with melatonin inhibited caspase activation and prevented reduction in MT1 receptors, suggesting that the protective effect of melatonin may be mediated through activation of its MT1 receptors.

Study of an Animal Model with Curcumin

Curcumin is a naturally occurring polyphenolic compound with the ability to cross the blood-brain barrier. The efficacy of curcumin in improving the symptoms was tested in a transgenic mouse model.

The results showed that Huntington's mice that had been fed with a curcumin-containing diet since conception showed decreased aggregates of HD protein and increased levels of dopamine and dopamine D1 receptor mRNAs in the striatal neurons, and had no abnormal pregnancies (Hickey et al. 2012).

Study of an Animal Model with Resveratrol

Using a rat HD model (3-NP-induced HD phenotype), it was demonstrated that the treatment of rats with resveratrol before and after 3-NP treatment reduced motor and cognitive deficits by reducing oxidaitve stress (Kumar et al. 2006).

Studies of an Animal Model with Ginkgo biloba *Extract and Olive Oil*

Pretreatment with *Ginkgo biloba* extract (EGb761) prevented 3-NP-induced motor deficits and reduced the levels of malondialdehyde (MDA) in the striatum of rats (Mahdy et al. 2011).

Treatment with extra-virgin olive oil prevented 3-NP-induced elevated levels of lipid peroxides and a depletion of glutathione in the striatum of rats (Tasset et al. 2011).

Study of an Animal Model with Probucol

Probucol, a cholesterol-lowering drug, is known to exhibit antioxidant activity. Using three Huntington's animal models, including quinolinic acid, 3-NP, and a combination of quinolinic acid and 3-NP-induced Huntington's disease, it was shown that treatment with probucol prevented free radical formation and lipid peroxidation in all animal models, but it did not protect against 3-NP-induced mitochondrial dysfunction (Colle et al. 2012). Treatment with sodium succinate protected striatal slices only against 3-NP-induced mitochondrial dysfunction. Treatment with an NMDA receptor antagonist MK-801 (also called dizocilpine) protected mitochondrial dysfunction in all Huntington's models used in this study.

These data suggest that a combination of NMDA receptor antagonists and an antioxidant may be more useful in reducing oxidatve stress and mitochondrial dysfunction than the individual agents.

Study of an Animal Model with B Vitamins

Nicotinamide, a water-soluble B_3 vitamin, is an inhibitor of histone deacetylase. Using a transgenic mouse model of Huntington's it was demonstrated that treatment with nicotinamide increased mRNA levels of BDNF and peroxisome proliferator-activated gamma receptor coactivator gamma-1alpha (PGC-1alpha). In addition, nicotinamide treatment enhanced the protein levels of BDNF and activation of PGC-1alpha in Huntington's mice. Furthermore, the above treatment improved motor function in Huntington's mice even though there was no reduction in the levels of HD protein aggregates in the striatum or weight loss (Hathorn, Snyder-Keller, and Messer 2011). Thus, vitamin B_3 may be of some value in improving motor function in the animal model.

Study of an Animal Model with Growth Factors

Immortalized nerve cells can grow indefinitely in petri dishes, but they do not produce cancer. This type of nerve cell, obtained from the striatum and expressing wild-type Huntington protein, acted as a normal control, whereas the same cell line expressing HD protein acted as a model for Huntington's disease. Using these cell lines the efficacy of various growth factors such as fetal and postnatal glia-condition medium (GCM), beta-fibroblastic growth factor (bFGF), brain-derived neurotrophic factor (BDNF), and glia-cell-derived neurotrophic factor (GDNF)—in protecting neurons against H_2O_2-, glutamate-, and 3-NP-induced toxicity—was evaluated. The results showed that GCM was most effective in protecting nerve cells expressing HD protein against the above neurotoxins. Fetal GCM also reduced the caspases fragmentation of the protein PARP, the expression of heat shock protein-70 (Hsp-70), accumulation of reactive oxygen species (ROS), and polyubiquitinated proteins (Ruiz et al. 2012). Thus, treatment with certain growth factors may be useful in reducing some symptoms.

The use of a single antioxidant cannot optimally suppress oxidative stress and chronic inflammation, because it cannot increase the levels of antioxidant enzymes as well as all dietary and endogenous antioxidants in the body. Therefore, the use of a single antioxidant produced minimal benefit even in animal models.

Studies of an Animal Model with Nrf2

Earlier we saw that increased oxidative stress and chronic inflammation play an important role in the development and progression of Parkinson's disease in humans. The same is true for Huntington's. The fact that increased levels of chronic oxidative stress are found in patients with Huntington's suggests that the Nrf2-ARE pathway responsible for increasing the levels of antioxidant enzymes has become unresponsive to ROS in this disease.

Treatment with quinolinic acid (an agonist of the N-methy-d-aspartate receptor) of slices from the rodent striatum induced degenerative changes in the neurons similar to those found in the brain neurons of Huntington's patients, which had been altered by increasing oxidative stress. Treatment of rodents (mice and rats) with quinolinic acid activated Nrf2, which increased phase-2-detoxifying enzymes and reduced oxidative damage (Colin-Gonzalez et al. 2014).

Neurons from the striatum-expressing HD gene (STHdh-Q111/Q111 cells) and neurons expressing the wild-type (normal) Huntington gene (STHdh-Q7/Q7 cell) were used to investigate the effect of the HD gene on mitochondrial function and oxidative stress. The results showed that neurons expressing HD genes had more fragmented mitochondria and more oxidative stress than did neurons expressing the wild-type Huntington gene. In addition, neurons expressing the HD gene had reduced activity of Nrf2, which increases the sensitivity of neurons to oxidative stress and mitochondrial dysfunction (Jin et al. 2013).

In a rat model induced by 3-nitropropionic acid (3-NP), the levels of Nrf2 were reduced in both the cytoplasm and the nucleus. Transcranial magnetic stimulation (TMS) is a noninvasive technique used in the treatment of different neuropsychiatric and neurodegenerative diseases. TMS treatment increased the levels of Nrf2 in the cytoplasm and the nucleus in a rat model (Tasset et al. 2013).

These studies suggest that activation of the Nrf2-ARE pathway may be useful in reducing the risk of developing Huntington's and helpful in limiting its progression.

Similarly to Parkinson's disease, the following groups of agents in combination may be useful in reducing the development and progression of Huntington's disease in humans.

1. **All antioxidants reduce varying levels of oxidative stress by directly scavenging free radicals:** Some examples are dietary antioxidants such as vitamin A, beta-carotene, vitamin C, and vitamin E and endogenous antioxidants such as glutathione, alpha-lipoic acid, and coenzyme Q10.

2. **Antioxidants that can reduce oxidative stress by activating the Nrf2-ARE pathway without ROS stimulation:** Some examples are the organosulfur compound sulforaphane found in cruciferous vegetables, kavalactones found in kava shrubs, and Puerarin, a major flavonoid from the root of *Pueraria lobata* (Wruck et al. 2008; Bergstrom et al. 2011; Zou et al. 2013). In addition, genistein and vitamin E (Xi et al. 2012), coenzyme Q10 (Choi et al. 2009), alpha-lipoic acid (Suh et al. 2004), curcumin (Trujillo et al. 2013), resveratrol (Steele et al. 2013; Kode et al. 2008), omega-3 fatty acids (Gao et al. 2007; Saw et al. 2013), and n-acetylcysteine (NAC) (Ji et al. 2010).

3. **Antioxidant compound that activates Nrf2 by a ROS-dependent mechanism:** L-carnitine activates Nrf2 without the need for ROS stimulation (Zambrano etal. 2013) probably by generating transient ROS.

A combination of selected agents from the above groups may optimally reduce oxidative stress, and thereby may reduce or delay the risk of developing Huntington's, and in combination with standard therapy, may improve the management of this disease.

HOW TO REDUCE CHRONIC INFLAMMATION AND GLUTAMATE

As with Parkinson's disease (and as discussed in chapter 5), some individual antioxidants from the above groups have been shown to reduce chronic inflammation (Abate et al. 2000; Devaraj et al. 2007; Fu et al. 2008; Lee et al. 2007; Peairs and Rankin 2008; Rahman et al. 2008; Suzuki, Aggarwal, and Packer 1992; Zhu et al. 2008) and prevent the release (Barger et al. 2007) and toxicity (Schubert, Kimura, and Maher 1992; Sandhu et al. 2003) of glutamate. Thus (and again, as with Parkinson's), a combination of selected agents from the above groups may optimally reduce chronic inflammation and release of glutamate and its toxicity and thereby may reduce the risk of developing Huntington's disease. Together with standard therapy, some of these agents in combination may improve its management.

PROBLEMS OF USING A SINGLE NUTRIENT

Some studies showed minimal beneficial effects of single antioxidants, B vitamins, or certain polyphenolic compounds alone in animal models. Only one study with vitamin E in human Huntington's showed no effect in patients, although minimal benefit was observed in patients with an early phase of the disease. The fact that patients have a high internal oxidative environment suggests that the administration of a single antioxidant would result in the oxidation of the administered antioxidant. As we have established and as is well known, an oxidized antioxidant acts as a prooxidant (like a free radical), which may not produce beneficial clinical outcomes. On the contrary, an oxidized antioxidant is likely to increase the progression of Huntington's after long-term consumption.

As we have established in chapter 5 in our discussion of Parkinson's disease, studies that have been undertaken on other chronic diseases using a single antioxidant produced conflicting results. This has led to my recommendation that a combination of micronutrients should be used to mitigate the risk of developing both Huntington's and Parkinson's disease and to enhance the efficacy of standard therapy in the management of both of these neurological conditions.

RATIONALE FOR USING MULTIPLE ANTIOXIDANTS*

In chapter 5, pertaining to Parkinson's disease, we discussed the mechanisms of action of antioxidants as part of a larger discussion about the best combination of micronutrients to select in combatting that disease. All of that rather long conversation is also applicable to Huntington's, so we have repeated the same information here.

In selecting micronutrients to include in the formula, it's important to note that the mechanisms of action of antioxidants in the proposed formulation are in part different. Their distribution in various organs and cells, their affinity to various types of free radicals, and their biological half-lives are different. For example, beta-carotene (BC) is more effective in scavenging oxygen radicals than most other antioxidants. Beta-carotene can perform certain biological functions that cannot be produced by vitamin A, and vitamin A can perform certain biological functions that cannot be performed by beta-carotene. It has been reported that BC treatment enhances the expression of the connexin gene, which codes for a gap junction protein in mammalian fibroblasts in culture, whereas vitamin A treatment does not produce such an effect. Vitamin A can induce differentiation in certain normal cells

---

*The references for this section are described in a review (Prasad, Cole, and Prasad 2002).

and cancer cells, whereas BC and other carotenoids do not. Thus, BC and vitamin A have, in part, different functions in the body.

The gradient of oxygen pressure varies within the cells. Some antioxidants, such as vitamin E, are more effective as scavengers of free radicals in an environment characterized by reduced oxygen pressure, whereas BC and vitamin A are more effective in an environment featuring higher atmospheric pressure.

Cells are made up of water and some fat. Cellular components are distributed in the water and fat of the cells. Vitamin C is necessary to protect cellular components in the water portion of the cells, whereas carotenoids, vitamin A, and vitamin E protect cellular components in the fat portion of the cells. Vitamin C also plays an important role in maintaining cellular levels of vitamin E by recycling the oxidized form of vitamin E (which acts as a prooxidant) to the reduced form of vitamin E (which acts as an antioxidant).

The *form* of vitamin E used is also an important consideration when devising a suitable micronutrient preparation. It has been established that d-alpha-tocopheryl succinate (vitamin E succinate) is the most effective form of vitamin E both in vitro and in vivo. This form of vitamin E is more soluble than alpha-tocopherol and enters cells more readily; therefore, it is expected to cross the blood-brain barrier in greater amounts than alpha-tocopherol.

We have reported that an oral ingestion of alpha-tocopheryl succinate (800 IU per day) in humans increased the plasma levels of not only alpha-tocopherol but also of vitamin E succinate, suggesting that a portion of vitamin E succinate can be absorbed from the intestinal tract before conversion to alpha-tocopherol. This observation is important, because the conventional assumption based on studies of rodents has been that esterified forms of vitamin E, such as alpha-tocopheryl succinate, alpha-tocopheryl nicotinate, and alpha-tocopheryl acetate, can be absorbed from the intestinal tract only after they are converted to the alpha-tocopherol form. Our preliminary data showed that this assumption may not be true for the absorption of vitamin E succinate in humans, provided that the pool of alpha-tocopherol in the blood is saturated.

Glutathione, which is an endogenous antioxidant, is effective in destroying H_2O_2 and superoxide anion (a form of free radical). However, oral supplementation with glutathione failed to significantly increase the plasma levels of glutathione in humans, suggesting that glutathione is completely destroyed in the intestine. Therefore, I propose to utilize n-acetylcysteine (NAC) and alpha-lipoic acid, which increase the cellular levels of glutathione by different mechanisms in a micronutrient preparation.

Coenzyme Q10 is another endogenous antioxidant that may have some potential value in the prevention and improved treatment of HD. Coenzyme Q10 administration has been shown to improve clinical symptoms in patients with mitochondrial encephalomyopathies (Chen, Huang, and Chu 1997). Given that mitochondrial dysfunction is associated with Huntington's and because coenzyme Q10 is needed for the generation of ATP by mitochondria, it is essential to add this antioxidant to a micronutrient preparation. A study has shown that coenzyme Q10 scavenges peroxy radicals faster than alpha-tocopherol and, like vitamin C, can convert oxidized vitamin E to the reduced form of vitamin E, which acts as an antioxidant.

Excessive amounts of glutamate release may cause degeneration of the nerve cells in Huntington's patients. Antioxidants reduced the release and toxicity of glutamate.

Nicotinamide (vitamin B_3) attenuated glutamate-induced toxicity in nerve cells. Nicotinamide is also an inhibitor of histone deacetylase activity and can restore memory deficits in neurodegenerative diseases, such as with Alzheimer's transgenic mice. Selenium is a cofactor of glutathione peroxidase, and Se-glutathione peroxidase acts as an antioxidant by increasing the intracellular level of glutathione.

In addition to dietary and endogenous antioxidants, B vitamins—especially high doses of nicotinamide (a form of vitamin B_3)—should be added to a multiple micronutrient preparation. B vitamins are essential for normal brain function. Omega-3 fatty acids were added because most clinical studies show some benefits to patients in another neurodegenerative disease—Alzheimer's.

Two recent clinical studies showed that supplementation with multiple vitamin preparations reduced cancer incidence by 10 percent in men (Gaziano et al. 2012) and improved clinical outcomes in patients with HIV/AIDS who were not taking medication (Baum et al. 2013).

CAN HUNTINGTON'S DISEASE BE PREVENTED OR DELAYED?

It's often believed that familial neurodegenerative diseases (derived from a family history of same) cannot be prevented or delayed by any pharmacological and/or physiological means. Laboratory experiments on the genetic basis of another disease (cancer) in the *Drosophila melanogaster* (fruit fly) model show that it may be possible to prevent or at least delay the onset of the disease.

The gene HOP (TUM-1) is essential to the development of fruit flies. A mutation in this gene markedly increases the risk of developing a leukemia-like tumor in female flies (unpublished observation in collaboration with Dr. Bhattacharya et al. of NASA, Moffat Field, California). Proton radiation is a powerful cancer-causing agent. Whole-body irradiation with proton radiation dramatically increased the incidence of cancer in these irradiated flies compared to that of unirradiated flies.

The question arose as to whether a preparation of multiple antioxidants might reduce the incidence of cancer that is due to a specific gene defect. To test this possibility, a mixture of multiple dietary and endogenous antioxidants were fed to these flies through diet seven days before proton irradiation and continued throughout the experimental period of seven days. The results showed that antioxidant treatment before and after irradiation totally blocked the proton radiation–induced cancer in fruit flies. This finding on fruit flies is of particular interest, because to my knowledge this is the first demonstration in which the genetic basis of a disease can be prevented by supplementation with multiple antioxidants.

This observation made on fruit flies cannot readily be extrapolated to humans. It is unknown whether daily supplementation with multiple antioxidants in children carrying the HD gene can prevent or delay the onset of the disease. The results on fruit flies suggest that daily supplementation with the proposed preparation of micronutrients could potentially prevent or delay the onset of symptoms. A clinical study to test the effectiveness of the proposed strategies—among individuals who are carrying the HD gene but have not developed any symptoms of the disease—should be tested.

PREVENTION OF HUNTINGTON'S DISEASE IN HUMANS

The purpose of prevention is to prevent or delay the onset of Huntington's symptoms in individuals carrying the HD gene but have not developed any symptoms of the disease. To develop prevention strategies it is essential to identify biochemical defects that initiate degeneration of nerve cells in the brain. Increased oxidative stress is one of the earliest biochemical defects in the initiation of damage to the nerve cells. Chronic inflammation, which participates in degeneration of the nerve cells, occurs subsequent to increased oxidative stress. Therefore, reducing oxidative stress and chronic inflammation are one of the rational choices for the prevention of Huntington's disease.

RECOMMENDED MICRONUTRIENTS IN THE PREVENTION OF HUNTINGTON'S DISEASE

The selected combination of nontoxic agents includes vitamin A (retinyl palmitate), B vitamins with higher levels of vitamin B_3 (nicotinamide), vitamin C (calcium ascorbate), vitamin D, vitamin E (both d-alpha-tocopherol and d-alpha-tocopheryl succinate), natural mixed carotenoids, selenium, coenzyme Q10, alpha-lipoic acid, n-acetylcysteine (NAC), L-carnitine, omega-3 fatty acids, resveratrol, and curcumin. The combination of the above agents was selected because they would optimally reduce oxidative stress and chronic inflammation by activating the Nrf2-ARE pathway without ROS stimulation and by directly scavenging free radicals. The doses of all ingredients are listed in table 7.1 on page 152. The daily doses can be divided in two, half to be taken in the morning and half in the evening, preferably with a meal.

The above formulation is unique, and it has no iron, copper, manganese, or heavy metals (vanadium, zirconium, or molybdenum). Iron and copper were not added, because they're known to interact with vitamin C and generate excessive amounts of free radicals. In addition, iron and copper are absorbed more in the presence of antioxidants than in the absence of antioxidants. Therefore, it is possible that prolonged consumption of these trace minerals in the presence of antioxidants may increase the levels of free iron or copper stores in the body, because there are no significant mechanisms of excretion of iron among men of all ages and women after menopause. Increased stores of free iron or copper may increase the risk of some human chronic diseases including Huntington's.

Heavy metals were not added, because prolonged consumption of these metals may increase their levels in the body due to the fact that there is no significant mechanism for excretion of these metals from the body; high levels of them are considered neurotoxic. The effectiveness of the proposed micronutrient preparation on individuals carrying the HD gene but not manifesting any symptoms should be tested by a well-designed clinical study.

Please e-mail knprasad@comcast.net for information on purchasing the above formulation.

TABLE 7.1. INGREDIENTS OF A RECOMMENDED MICRONUTRIENT PREPARATION (DAILY DOSES) FOR HUNTINGTON'S DISEASE*

Vitamin A (retinyl palmitate)	3,000 IU
Natural Vitamin E	400 IU (d-alpha-tocopheryl succinate 400 IU) (d-alpha-tocopheryl acetate 100 IU)
Vitamin C (calcium ascorbate)	1,500 mg
Vitamin D_3 (cholecalciferol)	1,000 IU
Vitamin B_1 (thiamine mononitrate)	4 mg
Vitamin B_2 (riboflavin)	5 mg
Vitamin B_3 (nicotinamide)	150 mg
Vitamin B_6 (pyridoxine hydrochloride)	5 mg
Folic acid (as folate)	800 mcg
Vitamin B_{12} (methylcobalamln)	10 mcg
Biotin	200 mcg
Pantothenic acid (calcium pantothenate)	10 mg
Calcium citrate	250 mg
Magnesium citrate	125 mg
Zinc glycinate	15 mg
Selenium (seleno-L-methionine)	200 mcg
Chromium (as picolinate)	50 mcg
N-acetylcysteine (NAC)	proprietary amount[†]
Coenzyme Q10	proprietary amount
Alpha-lipoic acid	proprietary amount
L-carnitine	proprietary amount
Curcumin	proprietary amount
Resveratrol	proprietary amount
Omega-3 fatty acids	proprietary amount

*Daily doses are divided into two doses, half to be taken in the morning and half in the evening, preferably with a meal. Children age 5–12 who are asymptomatic should take 20 percent of the adult dose. Adolescents age 13–17 should take 40 percent of the adult dose.
†Total amount of proprietary active blend is 1,620 mg.

USING A DOSE SCHEDULE

Most clinical studies with antioxidants in chronic diseases have utilized a once-a-day dose schedule. Taking vitamins and antioxidants once a day can create large fluctuations of their levels in the body. This is due to the fact that the biological half-lives of vitamins and antioxidants vary markedly depending upon their lipid- or water-solubility. A twofold difference in the levels of vitamin E succinate can produce marked alterations in the expression profiles of several genes in nerve cells in culture. Therefore, taking a multiple vitamin preparation once a day may produce large fluctuations in the levels of micronutrients in the body, which could potentially cause genetic stress in the cells, which may compromise the effectiveness of the vitamin supplementation after long-term consumption. I recommend taking the proposed preparation of micronutrients twice a day to reduce fluctuations in the levels of gene expression in the body. Such a dose schedule may improve the effectiveness of the proposed micronutrient preparation in reducing the development of Huntington's disease.

CAN ANTIOXIDANTS BE TOXIC?

Antioxidants, B vitamins, and certain polyphenolic compounds (curcumin and resveratrol) used in the proposed micronutrient preparation are considered safe. Antioxidants at doses higher than those that are recommended for the proposed micronutrient preparation have been consumed by the U.S. population for decades without significant toxicity being reported. However, a few of these antioxidants could produce harmful effects at certain high doses in some individuals when consumed daily for a long period of time.

For example, vitamin A at doses of 10,000 IU or more per day can cause birth defects in pregnant women, and beta-carotene at doses of 50 milligrams or more can produce bronzing of the skin that is reversible on discontinuation. Vitamin C as ascorbic acid at high doses (10 grams or more per day) can cause diarrhea in some individuals. Vitamin E at high doses (2,000 IU or more per day) can induce clotting defects after long-term consumption. Vitamin B_6 at high doses (50 milligrams or more per day) may produce peripheral neuropathy, and selenium at doses of 400 micrograms or more per day can cause skin and liver toxicity after long-term consumption. Coenzyme Q10 has no known toxicity, and recommended daily doses are 30 to 400 milligrams. N-acetylcysteine (NAC) doses of 250 to 1,500 milligrams, and alpha-lipoic acid doses of 600 milligrams are used in humans without toxicity at these doses. All ingredients present in the proposed micronutrient preparations are safe and are classified as food supplements. Therefore they don't require FDA approval for their use.

FURTHER THERAPY AND MEDICATION

Current treatment strategies for Huntington's disease are based on improving the symptoms rather than the causes of the disease. At present no drug treatment can alter the course of this disease in people. And although a combination of medications, psychotherapy, speech therapy, and physical therapy may reduce some symptoms, it cannot alter the course of the disease. The current treatment approaches are described here. They include various types of therapy as well as different medications.*

Psychotherapy
Psychotherapy may be provided by a psychiatrist, psychologist, or social worker and is beneficial in helping people afflicted with Huntington's manage any behavioral problems they may be experiencing. It may also be useful in managing expectations during the progression of the disease and facilitating effective communication among family members. This form of therapy is used in combination with drug therapy.

---

*The information about the different drugs is derived from publications of the Mayo Clinic Foundation for Medical Education and Research.

Speech Therapy

HD can markedly impair control of the muscles of the mouth and throat that are essential for speaking, eating, and swallowing. A speech therapist can help to improve a person's ability to speak clearly and to use communication devices correctly. This therapy is used in combination with other therapies.

Physical Therapy

Physical therapy may improve motor function. A physical therapist can help the afflicted person learn how to exercise safely and correctly to enhance muscle strength, flexibility, balance, and coordination. Exercise can help in maintaining mobility as long as possible and may reduce the risk of falling. The physical therapist can also provide instruction on the appropriate posture and the use of supports to improve posture, which may reduce the severity of some movement disorders. For those patients who may require a wheelchair or a walker, a physical therapist can teach them to use these devices correctly. Physical activity is essential for Huntington's patients, but this should be performed under the supervision of a physical therapist and/or professional caregiver.

Therapy Pertaining to Weight Loss

Weight loss is one of the features of Huntington's disease, which may be caused in part by the afflicted person's difficulty in swallowing. People with Huntington's typically take a long time to consume their food and may run the risk of choking on it. Patients should consume enough calories to maintain their body weight. Caregivers are often trained how to deal with problems related to food consumption. It is also important that patients be sufficiently hydrated at all times.

Antidepressants

Commonly used antidepressants include escitalopram (Lexapro), fluoxetine (Prozac, Sarafem), and sertraline (Zoloft). (These drugs may also be useful in treating obsessive-compulsive disorder.) Some side effects may include nausea, diarrhea, insomnia, and sexual problems.

Mood-Stabilizing Drugs

Mood-stabilizing drugs for persons with Huntington's include lithium (Lithobid) and anticonvulsants, such as valporic acid (Depakene), divalproex (Depakote), and lamotrigine (Lamictal), which are also useful in the treatment of highs and lows associated with bipolar disorder. Common side effects include weight gain, tremor, and gastrointestinal problems. Periodic blood tests are needed because of the toxicity of lithium on the thyroid and kidneys.

Drugs Affecting Movement

Given that movement disorder is the major symptom of Huntington's, the primary purpose of treatment has been to reduce movement disorders through the use of appropriate medication. To this end, different classes of drugs have been used to improve motor function. Tetrabenazine (Xenazine) is an FDA-approved drug used to suppress the chorea (jerking movements) associated with the disease. Although this drug improves movement disorders, the risk of serious side effects include the risk of triggering depression or, if preexisting, of making the depression worse. This drug may also exacerbate other psychiatric problems, insomnia, drowsiness, nausea, and restlessness.

Antipsychotic Drugs

Antipsychotic drugs such as haloperidol (Haldol) and clozapine can suppress chorea, but they can worsen involuntary contractions (dystonia) and muscle rigidity.

Antiseizure and Antianxiety Drugs

Other drugs—including antiseizure drugs such as clonazepam (Klonopin) and antianxiety medications such as diazepam (Valium)—can suppress chorea, dystonia, and muscle rigidity. These drugs can also alter consciousness and induce addiction and dependency.

Limitations of Current Medications

The currently used medications do not affect oxidative stress and chronic inflammation. Consequently, neurons continue to die and the beneficial effects of the drugs don't last long.

Clinical Studies of Additional Medications

In a clinical study of six Huntington's patients, the effectiveness of aripiprazole (AP), a dopamine D2 receptor partial agonist that is used to reduce schizophrenic symptoms, was compared with tetrabenazine (TBZ). TBZ, which depletes dopamine, is used to treat hyperkinesia (chorea), motor function, and functional disability. The results showed that both drugs reduce chorea in a similar manner; however, AP caused less sedation and sleepiness than TBZ (Brusa et al. 2009). The sample size of this study is too small to make any valid conclusions. It's interesting to note that two drugs that have an opposite effect on the level of dopamine were used in this study.

In a randomized, double-blind, placebo-controlled trial involving multicenters of thirty-two European countries, the effectiveness of pridopidine, a dopaminergic stabilizer, was evaluated on motor function in Huntington's patients. The results showed that this drug did not affect non-motor functions but produced some improvements in motor function (de Yebenes et al. 2011). The drug at the dose of 90 milligrams per day was considered safe.

A similar study with pridopidine was performed utilizing outpatient neurological clinics at twenty-seven sites in the United States and Canada. The study was performed on patients receiving 20 milligrams (N = 56), 45 milligrams (N = 55), 90 milligrams (N = 58), or placebo (N = 58) for a period of twelve weeks. The results showed that pridopidine treatment at a dose of 90 milligrams per day may improve some motor functions in patients (Investigators 2013).

RECOMMENDED MICRONUTRIENTS IN COMBINATION WITH STANDARD THERAPY

In addition to increased oxidative stress, chronic inflammation, and mitochondrial dysfunction, glutamate is also released in patients with established Huntington's symptoms. Glutamate is toxic to the nerve cells. Antioxidants prevent the release and toxicity of glutamate (Barger et al. 2007; Schubert, Kimura, and Maher 1992). Therefore, the proposed micronutrients (table 7.1 on page 152) for prevention can also be used in combination with standard therapy for those individuals who have established symptoms of Huntington's disease. For those symptomatic patients who cannot swallow food, micronutrients from the capsules can be mixed with a liquid such as juice.

The doses and dose schedule of the proposed micronutrient preparation are the same as what is recommended for prevention. A clinical study using the proposed strategies on patients who are at the various stages of the disease and taking medication should be initiated.

The daily recommended doses of the proposed micronutrient preparation for adults (eighteen years or older) are presented in table 7.1. Again, daily doses are to be divided in two, with half to be taken in the morning and half in the evening, preferably with a meal. Also provided are dose schedules for children and adolescents; see table 7.1 footnote.

DIET AND LIFESTYLE RECOMMENDATIONS

For asymptomatic individuals carrying the HD gene I recommend daily consumption of a low-fat, high-fiber diet with plenty of fruit (especially grapes and berries) and leafy vegetables. It's also advisable to avoid an excessive intake of carbohydrates and proteins. Whenever oil is used for cooking, virgin olive oil is preferred. For non-vegetarians, fish (especially salmon) twice a week and chicken (or other meat, not more than 4 ounces per meal) is recommended. For vegetarians an increased intake of lima beans and soy products is recommended. Certain spices and herbs such as turmeric, cinnamon, garlic, and ginger can be added to the preparation of vegetables or meat. These spices and herbs have exhibited antioxidant and anti-inflammatory activities.

For individuals with established Huntington's disease, changes in lifestyle recommendations include maintaining normal weight by losing weight if one needs to (especially if one is obese), increasing physical activity, ceasing the smoking of tobacco, reducing stress (by way of a vacation and the practice of yoga and/or meditation), and performing moderate exercise four or five times a week. Moderate exercise includes walking twenty to twenty-five minutes per day at least five days per week, or using a treadmill (twenty-five minutes at a moderate speed), and weight lifting for thirty minutes three to four times a week. The level of exercise depends on the age of the individual, given that younger individuals can usually do more strenuous exercise than can older individuals.

CONCLUDING REMARKS

Despite the identification of various biochemical defects such as increased oxidative stress, mitochondrial dysfunction, and chronic inflammation, all of which participate in the development of Huntington's disease, no prevention strategies to prevent or delay the onset of symptoms are available. Based on known biochemical defects, reducing oxidative stress and chronic inflammation appear to be one of rational choices for the prevention of Huntington's disease or delaying its onset. Reduction of oxidative stress and chronic inflammation can be achieved by elevating antioxidant enzymes as well as all dietary and endogenous antioxidants. The use of a single antioxidant cannot achieve this same goal.

Unfortunately, most studies have utilized a single antioxidant in animal models. Only one study with vitamin E has been performed in humans. These studies have yielded minimal or no benefits in improving Huntington's symptoms. I have proposed a preparation of micronutrients that contains multiple dietary and endogenous antioxidants, vitamin D, all of the B vitamins (with high doses of vitamin B_3), selenium, certain polyphenolic compounds (curcumin and resveratrol), and omega-3 fatty acids, which would meet the above-referenced targeted goals. The effectiveness of this approach should be tested by clinical studies.

In determining a strategy of treatment, the symptoms are focused on rather than what is causing Huntington's, and thus the primary purpose of treatment has typically been to improve the symptoms as much as possible. Movement-disorder drugs, antipsychotic drugs, and mood-stabilizing drugs that are used in this regard are not very effective and have serious side effects to boot. Therapeutic modalities include psychotherapy, speech therapy, and physical therapy, which do nothing to address the levels oxidative stress and chronic inflammation that are the hallmarks of Huntington's disease. As a result, the disease progresses in a routine fashion, and, given that there is no cure for it, it eventually proves fatal.

The micronutrient preparation that I propose, in combination with standard therapy, may reduce the progression of the disease and improve its management. The effectiveness of the proposed approach should be tested by clinical studies, but until such time as that should come to pass, it's suggested that individuals carrying the HD gene who have not yet developed any symptoms of the disease, and those with established Huntington's symptoms, should adopt the proposed recommendations in consultation with a neurologist and/or a primary care physician.

Values of Recommended Dietary Allowances (RDA)/ Dietary Reference Intakes (DRI)

Note to the Reader: All of the information contained in this appendix, including the tables, is from my book *Fighting Cancer with Vitamins and Antioxidants,* coauthored with my son K. C. Prasad, M.S., M.D., and published by Healing Arts Press in 2011.

■ ■ ■

Sufficient changes in nutritional guidelines have occurred since World War II due to increased knowledge of nutrition and health. The nutritional guidelines referred to as Recommended Dietary Allowances (RDAs) were first established in 1941. The Food and Nutrition Board of the United States subsequently revise these guidelines every five to ten years.

RDA (DRI)

RDA refers to the value of the daily dietary intake level of a nutrient considered sufficient to meet the requirements of 97 to 98 percent of healthy individuals of different ages and genders. Because of the rapid growth of research on the role of nutrients in human health, the Food and Nutrition Board of the Institute of Medicine (IOM) of the United States in collaboration with Health Canada updated the values of RDAs and renamed them Dietary Reference Intakes (DRIs) in 1998. Since then DRI values have been used by both the United States and Canada. The DRI values of selected nutrients are listed in tables A.1 to A.21. The DRI values are not currently used in nutrition labeling; the RDA values of nutrients continue to be used for this purpose. The DRI values for carotenoids, alpha-lipoic acid, n-acetylcysteine, coenzyme Q10, and L-carnitine have not been determined.

ADEQUATE INTAKE (AI)

Adequate intake refers to the value of a nutrient for which no RDA has been established, but the value established may be sufficient for everyone in the demographic group.

TOLERABLE UPPER INTAKE LEVEL (UL)

The tolerable upper intake level is the maximum level of daily nutrient intake that is likely to pose no risk of adverse health effects. The UL value represents total intake of a nutrient from food, water, and supplements.

RELATIONSHIP BETWEEN RECOMMENDED DIETARY ALLOWANCE VALUES AND OPTIMAL HEALTH

RDA values of nutrients are expected to be adequate for individuals for normal growth and survival; however, the values of micronutrients needed for prevention or improved management of human diseases are not known at this time. The data on doses obtained from the use of a single micronutrient in the prevention or treatment of neurological conditions should not be extrapolated to the doses of the same micronutrient present in a multiple micronutrient preparation.

RDA/DRI values of micronutrients are sufficient for normal growth and survival, but they are not adequate for prevention or improved treatment of human diseases. To evaluate the dosage of micronutrients in any multivitamin preparation for the prevention or improved treatment of neurological conditions, it is essential to have sufficient knowledge of the RDA values of the micronutrients as found in the next section of this book.

CONCLUDING REMARKS

The initial nutritional guidelines, Recommended Dietary Allowances (RDAs), have been replaced by Dietary Reference Intakes (DRIs) and are currently used in the United States and Canada. The DRI values of nutrients are sufficient for the growth and development of 97 to 98 percent of healthy individuals. The DRI values for carotenoids, alpha-lipoic acid, n-acetylcysteine, coenzyme Q10, and L-carnitine have not been determined. The optimal values needed for the prevention or improved management of Parkinson's and Huntington's disease are not known. Both preventive and therapeutic doses of micronutrients are higher than their RDA values.

TABLE A.1. DIETARY REFERENCE
INTAKES (DRI) OF ANTIOXIDANT VITAMIN A

Age	RDA/AI*	UL
	µg/d (IU/d)	µg/d (IU/d)
Infants		
0–6 mo	400 (1,200 IU)*	600 (1,800 IU)
7–12 mo	500 (1,500 IU)*	600 (1,800 IU)
Children		
1–3 y	300 (900 IU)	600 (1,800 IU)
4–8 y	400 (1,200 IU)	900 (2,700 IU)
Males		
9–13 y	600 (1,800 IU)	1,700 (5,100 IU)
14–18 y	900 (2,700 IU)	2,800 (8,400 IU)
19 y and up	900 (2,700 IU)	3,000 (9,000 IU)
Females		
9–13 y	600 (1,800 IU)	1,700 (5,100 IU)
14–18 y	700 (2,100 IU)	2,800 (8,400 IU)
19 y and up	700 (2,100 IU)	3,000 (9,000 IU)
Pregnancy		
under 18 y	750 (2,250 IU)	2,800 (8,400 IU)
19–50 y	770 (2,310 IU)	3,000 (9,000 IU)
Lactation		
under 18 y	1,200 (3,600 IU)	2,800 (8,400 IU)
19–50 y	1,300 (3,900 IU)	3,000 (9,000 IU)

1 µg of retinol equals 1 µg of RAE (retinol activity equivalent); 1 IU of retinol equals 0.3 µg of retinol; and 2 µg of beta-carotene equals 1 µg of retinol.

RDA = Recommended Dietary Allowances
*AI = Adequate Intake
UL = Tolerable Upper Intake Value
µg = microgram; d = day

The values are adapted and summarized from the table of the Dietary Reference Intakes (DRI) published by www.nap.edu. (Search on "Food and Nutrition" and you will find information about DRI.)

TABLE A.2. DIETARY REFERENCE INTAKES (DRI) OF ANTIOXIDANT VITAMIN C

Age	RDA/AI*	UL
	mg/d	mg/d
Infants		
0–6 mo	40*	ND
7–12 mo	50*	ND
Children		
1–3 y	15	400
4–8 y	25	650
Males		
9–13 y	45	1,200
14–18 y	75	1,800
19 y and up	90	2,000
Females		
9–13 y	45	1,200
14–18 y	65	1,800
19 y and up	75	2,000

RDA = Recommended Dietary Allowances
*AI = Adequate Intake
UL = Tolerable Upper Intake Value
mg = microgram; d = day
ND = not determined

The values are adapted and summarized from the table of the Dietary Reference Intakes (DRI) published by www.nap.edu.

TABLE A.3. DIETARY REFERENCE
INTAKES (DRI) OF ANTIOXIDANT VITAMIN E

Age	RDA/AI*	UL
	mg/d (IU/d)	mg/d (IU/d)
Infants		
0–6 mo	4 (6 IU)*	ND
7–12 mo	5 (7.5 IU)*	ND
Children		
1–3 y	6 (9 IU)	200 (30 IU)
4–8 y	7 (10.6 IU)	300 (45 IU)
Males		
9–13 y	11 (16.7 IU)	600 (90 IU)
14–18 y	15 (22.8 IU)	800 (120 IU)
19 y and up	15 (22.8 IU)	1,000 (150 IU)
Females		
9–13 y	11 (16.7 IU)	600 (90 IU)
14–18 y	15 (22.8 IU)	800 (120 IU)
19 y and up	15 (22.8 IU)	1,000 (150 IU)
Pregnancy		
under 18 y	15 (22.8 IU)	800 (120 IU)
19–50 y	15 (22.8 IU)	1,000 (150 IU)
Lactation		
under 18 y	19 (28.9 IU)	800 (120 IU)
19–50 y	19 (28.9 IU)	1,000 (150 IU)

RDA = Recommended Dietary Allowances
*AI = Adequate Intake
UL = Tolerable Upper Intake Value
ND = not determined
mg = milligram; d = day
1 IU of vitamin E equals 0.66 mg of d- and 0.45 mg of
    dl-alpha-tocopherol.

The values are adapted and summarized from the tables of the Dietary Reference Intakes (DRI)
published by www.nap.edu.

TABLE A.4. DIETARY REFERENCE
INTAKES (DRI) OF VITAMIN D

Age	RDA/AI*	UL
	µg/d (IU/d)	µg/d (IU/d)
Infants		
0–12 mo	5 (200 IU)*	25 (1,000 IU)
Children		
1–8 y	5 (200 IU)*	50 (2,000 IU)
Males		
9–50 y	5 (200 IU)*	50 (2,000 IU)
50–70 y	10 (400 IU)*	50 (2,000 IU)
over 70 y	15 (600 IU)*	50 (2,000 IU)
Females		
9–50 y	5 (200 IU)*	50 (2,000 IU)
50–70 y	10 (400 IU)*	50 (2,000 IU)
under 70 y	15 (600 IU)*	50 (2,000 IU)
Pregnancy		
18–50 y	5 (200 IU)*	50 (2,000 IU)
Lactation		
18–50 y	5 (200 IU)*	50 (2,000 IU)

RDA = Recommended Dietary Allowances
*AI = Adequate Intake
UL = Tolerable Upper Intake Value
µg = microgram; d = day
1 µg of cholecalciferol equals 40 IU (international
    unit) of vitamin D.

The values are adapted and summarized from the tables of the Dietary Reference Intakes (DRI)
published by www.nap.edu.

TABLE A.5. DIETARY REFERENCE
INTAKES (DRI) OF VITAMIN B₁ (THIAMINE)

Age	RDA/AI*	UL
	mg/d	mg/d
Infants		
0–6 mo	0.2*	ND
7–12 mo	0.3*	ND
Children		
1–3 y	0.5	ND
4–8 y	0.6	ND
Males		
9–13 y	0.9	ND
14 y and up	1.2	ND
Females		
9–13 y	0.9	ND
14–18 y	1.0	ND
19 y and up	1.1	ND
Pregnancy		
18–50 y	1.4	ND
Lactation		
18–50 y	1.4	ND

RDA = Recommended Dietary Allowances
*AI = Adequate Intake
UL = Tolerable Upper Intake Value
ND = not determined
mg = milligram; d = day

The values are adapted and summarized from the tables of the Dietary Reference Intakes (DRI) published by www.nap.edu.

TABLE A.6. DIETARY REFERENCE
INTAKES (DRI) OF VITAMIN B$_2$ (RIBOFLAVIN)

Age	RDA/AI*	UL
	mg/d	mg/d
Infants		
0–6 mo	0.3*	ND
7–12 mo	0.4*	ND
Children		
1–3 y	0.5	ND
4–8 y	0.6	ND
Males		
9–13 y	0.9	ND
14 y and up	13	ND
Females		
9–13 y	0.9	ND
14–18 y	1.0	ND
19 y and up	1.1	ND
Pregnancy		
18–50 y	1.4	ND
Lactation		
18–50 y	1.6	ND

RDA = Recommended Dietary Allowances
*AI = Adequate Intake
UL = Tolerable Upper Intake Value
ND = not determined
mg = milligram; d = day

The values are adapted and summarized from the table of the Dietary Reference Intakes (DRI) published by www.nap.edu.

TABLE A.7. DIETARY REFERENCE
INTAKES (DRI) OF VITAMIN B$_6$

Age	RDA/AI*	UL
	mg/d	mg/d
Infants		
0–6 mo	0.1*	ND
7–12 mo	0.3*	ND
Children		
1–3 y	0.5	30
4–8 y	0.6	40
Males		
9–13 y	1.0	60
14–50 y	1.3	80
50–70 y and up	1.7	100
Females		
9–13 y	1.0	60
14–18 y	1.2	80
19–30 y	1.3	100
50 y and up	1.5	100
Pregnancy		
under 18 y	1.9	80
19–50 y	1.9	100
Lactation		
under 18 y	2.0	80
19–50 y	2.0	100

RDA = Recommended Dietary Allowances
*AI = Adequate Intake
UL = Tolerable Upper Intake Value
ND = not determined
mg = milligram; d = day

The values are adapted and summarized from the table of the Dietary Reference Intakes (DRI) published by www.nap.edu.

TABLE A.8. DIETARY REFERENCE INTAKES (DRI) OF VITAMIN B₁₂ (COBALAMIN)

Age	RDA/AI*	UL
	µg/d	µg/d
Infants		
0–6 mo	0.4*	ND
7–12 mo	0.5*	ND
Children		
1–3 y	0.9	ND
4–8 y	1.2	ND
Males		
9–13 y	1.08	ND
14 y and up	2.4	ND
Females		
9–13 y	1.8	ND
14 y and up	2.4	ND
Pregnancy		
18–50 y	2.6	ND
Lactation		
18–50 y	2.8	ND

RDA = Recommended Dietary Allowances
*AI = Adequate Intake
UL = Tolerable Upper Intake Value
ND = not determined
µg = microgram; d = day

The values are adapted and summarized from the table of the Dietary Reference Intakes (DRI) published by www.nap.edu.

TABLE A.9. DIETARY REFERENCE
INTAKES (DRI) OF VITAMIN B₅ (PANTOTHENIC ACID)

Age	RDA/AI*	UL
	mg/d	mg/d
Infants		
0–6 mo	1.7*	ND
7–12 mo	1.8*	ND
Children		
1–3 y	2*	ND
4–8 y	2*	ND
Males		
9–13 y	4*	ND
14 y and up	5*	ND
Females		
9–13 y	4*	ND
14 y and up	5*	ND
Pregnancy		
18–50 y	6*	ND
Lactation		
18–50 y	7*	ND

RDA = Recommended Dietary Allowances
*AI = Adequate Intake
UL = Tolerable Upper Intake Value
ND = not determined
mg = milligram; d = day

The values are adapted and summarized from the table of the Dietary Reference Intakes (DRI) published by www.nap.edu.

TABLE A.10. DIETARY REFERENCE INTAKES (DRI) OF VITAMIN B$_3$ (NIACIN)

Age	RDA/AI*	UL
	mg/d	mg/d
Infants		
0–6 mo	2*	ND
7–12 mo	0.4*	ND
Children		
1–3 y	6.0	10
4–8 y	8.0	15
Males		
9–13 y	12	20
14–50 y	16	30
50 y and up	16	35
Females		
9–13 y	12	20
14–18 y	14	30
19 y and up	14	35
Pregnancy		
under 18 y	18	30
19–50 y	18	35
Lactation		
under 18 y	17	30
19–50 y	17	35

RDA = Recommended Dietary Allowances
*AI = Adequate Intake
UL = Tolerable Upper Intake Value
ND = not determined
mg = milligram; d = day

The values are adapted and summarized from the table of the Dietary Reference Intakes (DRI) published by www.nap.edu

TABLE A.11. DIETARY REFERENCE
INTAKES (DRI) OF VITAMIN B₉ (FOLATE)

Age	RDA/AI*	UL
	µg/d	µg/d
Infants		
0–6 mo	65*	ND
7–12 mo	80*	ND
Children		
1–3 y	150	300
4–8 y	200	400
Males		
9–13 y	300	600
14–18 y	400	800
19 y and up	400	1,000
Females		
9–13 y	300	600
14–18 y	400	800
19 y and up	400	1,000
Pregnancy		
under 18 y	600	800
19–50 y	600	1,000
Lactation		
under 18 y	500	800
19–50 y	500	1,000

RDA = Recommended Dietary Allowances
*AI = Adequate Intake
UL = Tolerable Upper Intake Value
ND = not determined
µg = microgram; d = day

The values are adapted and summarized from the table of the Dietary Reference Intakes (DRI) published by www.nap.edu.

TABLE A.12. DIETARY REFERENCE
INTAKES (DRI) OF MICRONUTRIENT BIOTIN

Age	RDA/AI*	UL
	µg/d	µg/d
Infants		
0–6 mo	0.5*	ND
7–12 mo	0.6*	ND
Children		
1–3 y	8*	ND
4–8 y	12*	ND
Males		
9–13 y	20	ND
14–18 y	25	ND
19 y and up	30	ND
Females		
9–13 y	20	ND
14–18 y	25	ND
19 y and up	30	ND
Pregnancy		
under 18 y	30*	ND
19–50 y	30*	ND
Lactation		
under 18 y	35*	ND
19–50 y	35*	ND

RDA = Recommended Dietary Allowances
*AI = Adequate Intake
UL = Tolerable Upper Intake Value
ND = not determined
µg = microgram; d = day

The values are adapted and summarized from the table of the Dietary Reference Intakes (DRI)
published by www.nap.edu.

TABLE A.13. DIETARY REFERENCE
INTAKES (DRI) OF MINERAL CALCIUM

Age	RDA/AI*	UL
	mg/d	mg/d
Infants		
0–6 mo	210*	ND
7–12 mo	270*	ND
Children		
1–3 y	500*	2,500
4–8 y	800*	2,500
Males		
9–18 y	1,300*	2,500
19–50 y	1,000*	2,500
51 y and up	1,200*	2,500
Females		
9–8 y	1,300*	2,500
19–50 y	1,000*	2,500
51 y and up	1,200*	2,500
Pregnancy		
under 18 y	1,300*	2,500
19–50 y	1,000*	2,500
Lactation		
under 18 y	1,300*	2,500
19–50 y	1,000*	2,500

RDA = Recommended Dietary Allowances
*AI = Adequate Intake
UL = Tolerable Upper Intake Value
ND = not determined
mg = milligram; d = day

The values are adapted and summarized from the table of the Dietary Reference Intakes (DRI) published by www.nap.edu.

TABLE A.14. DIETARY REFERENCE
INTAKES (DRI) OF MINERAL MAGNESIUM

Age	RDA/AI*	UL
	mg/d	mg/d
Infants		
0–6 mo	30*	ND
7–12 mo	75*	ND
Children		
1–3 y	80	65
4–8 y	130	110
Males		
9–13 y	240	350
14–18 y	410	350
19–30 y	400	350
31 y and up	420	350
Females		
9–13 y	240	350
14–18 y	360	350
31 y and up	320	350
Pregnancy		
under 18 y	400	350
19–30 y	350	350
31–50 y	360	350
Lactation		
under 18 y	360	350
31–50 y	320	350

RDA = Recommended Dietary Allowances
*AI = Adequate Intake
UL = Tolerable Upper Intake Value
ND = not determined
mg = milligram; d = day

The values are adapted and summarized from the table of the Dietary Reference Intakes (DRI)
published by www.nap.edu.

TABLE A.15. DIETARY REFERENCE
INTAKES (DRI) OF MINERAL MANGANESE

Age	RDA/AI*	UL
	mg/d	mg/d
Infants		
0–6 mo	0.003*	ND
7–12 mo	0.6*	ND
Children		
1–3 y	1.2*	2
4–8 y	1.5*	3
Males		
9–13 y	1.9*	6
14–18 y	2.2*	9
19 y and up	2.3*	11
Females		
9–13 y	1.6*	6
14–18 y	1.6*	9
19 y and up	1.8*	11
Pregnancy		
under 18 y	2.0*	9
19–50 y	2.0*	11
Lactation		
under 18 y	2.6*	9
19–50 y	2.6*	11

RDA = Recommended Dietary Allowances
*AI = Adequate Intake
UL = Tolerable Upper Intake Value
ND = not determined
mg = milligram; d = day

The values are adapted and summarized from the table of the Dietary Reference Intakes (DRI) published by www.nap.edu.

TABLE A.16. DIETARY REFERENCE INTAKES (DRI) OF MINERAL CHROMIUM

Age	RDA/AI*	UL
	µg/d	µg/d
Infants		
0–6 mo	0.2*	ND
7–12 mo	5.5*	ND
Children		
1–3 y	11*	ND
4–8 y	15*	ND
Males		
9–13 y	25*	ND
14–50 y	35*	ND
51 y and up	30*	ND
Females		
9–13 y	21*	ND
14–18 y	24*	ND
19–50 y	25*	ND
Pregnancy		
under 18 y	29*	ND
19–50 y	30*	ND
Lactation		
under 18 y	44*	ND
19–50 y	45*	ND

RDA = Recommended Dietary Allowances
*AI = Adequate Intake
UL = Tolerable Upper Intake Value
ND = not determined
µg = microgram; d = day

The values are adapted and summarized from the table of the Dietary Reference Intakes (DRI) published by www.nap.edu.

TABLE A.17. DIETARY REFERENCE INTAKES (DRI) OF MINERAL COPPER

Age	RDA/AI*	UL
	µg/d	µg/d
Infants		
0–6 mo	200*	ND
7–12 mo	220*	ND
Children		
1–3 y	340	1,000
4–8 y	440	3,000
Males		
9–13 y	700	5,000
14–18 y	890	8,000
19 y and up	900	10,000
Females		
9–13 y	700	5,000
14–18 y	890	8,000
19 y and up	900	10,000
Pregnancy		
under 18 y	1,000	8,000
19–50 y	1,000	10,000
Lactation		
under 18 y	1,300	8,000
19–50 y	1,300	10,000

RDA = Recommended Dietary Allowances
*AI = Adequate Intake
UL = Tolerable Upper Intake Value
ND = not determined
µg = microgram; d = day

The values are adapted and summarized from the table of the Dietary Reference Intakes (DRI) published by www.nap.edu.

TABLE A.18. DIETARY REFERENCE INTAKES (DRI) OF MINERAL IRON

Age	RDA/AI*	UL
	mg/d	mg/d
Infants		
0–6 mo	0.27*	40
7–12 mo	11	40
Children		
1–3 y	7	40
4–8 y	10	40
Males		
9–13 y	8	40
14–18 y	11	45
19 y and up	8	45
Females		
9–13 y	8	40
14–18 y	15	45
19–50 y	18	45
50 y and up	8	45
Pregnancy		
18–50 y	27	45
Lactation		
under 18 y	10	45
19–50 y	9	45

RDA = Recommended Dietary Allowances
*AI = Adequate Intake
UL = Tolerable Upper Intake Value
ND = not determined
mg = milligram; d = day

The values are adapted and summarized from the table of the Dietary Reference Intakes (DRI) published by www.nap.edu.

TABLE A.19. DIETARY REFERENCE
INTAKES (DRI) OF MINERAL SELENIUM

Age	RDA/AI*	UL
	µg/d	µg/d
Infants		
0–6 mo	15*	45
7–12 mo	20*	60
Children		
1–3 y	20	90
4–8 y	30	150
Males		
9–13 y	40	280
14 y and up	55	400
Females		
9–13 y	40	280
14 y and up	55	400
Pregnancy		
18–50 y	60	400
Lactation		
18–50 y	70	400

RDA = Recommended Dietary Allowances
*AI = Adequate Intake
UL = Tolerable Upper Intake Value
ND = not determined
µg = microgram; d = day

The values are adapted and summarized from the table of the Dietary Reference Intakes (DRI) published by www.nap.edu.

TABLE A.20. DIETARY REFERENCE
INTAKES (DRI) OF MINERAL PHOSPHORUS

Age	RDA/AI*	UL
	mg/d	mg/d
Infants		
0–6 mo	100*	ND
7–12 mo	275*	ND
Children		
1–3 y	460	3,000
4–8 y	500	3,000
Males		
9–18 y	1,250	4,000
19–70 y	700	4,000
70 y and up	700	3,000
Females		
9–18 y	1,250	4,000
19–70 y	700	4,000
70 y and up	700	3,000
Pregnancy		
under 18 y	1,250	3,500
19–50 y	700	3,500
Lactation		
under 18 y	1,250	4,000
19–50 y	700	4,000

RDA = Recommended Dietary Allowances
*AI = Adequate Intake
UL = Tolerable Upper Intake Value
ND = not determined
mg = milligram; d = day

The values are adapted and summarized from the table of the Dietary Reference Intakes (DRI)
published by www.nap.edu.

TABLE A.21. DIETARY REFERENCE INTAKES (DRI) OF MINERAL ZINC

Age	RDA/AI*	UL
	mg/d	mg/d
Infants		
0–6	2*	4
7–12 mo	3	5
Children		
1–3 y	3	7
4–8 y	5	12
Males		
9–13 y	8	23
14–18 y	11	34
19 y and up	11	40
Females		
9–13 y	8	23
14–18 y	9	34
19 y and up	8	40
Pregnancy		
under 18 y	12	34
19–50 y	11	40
Lactation		
under 18 y	13	34
19–50 y	12	40

RDA = Recommended Dietary Allowances
*AI = Adequate Intake
UL = Tolerable Upper Intake Value
ND = not determined
mg = milligram; d = day

The values are adapted and summarized from the table of the Dietary Reference Intakes (DRI) published by www.nap.edu.

TABLE A.22. CALORIE CONTENT
OF SELECTED FOODS

Food	Portion size	Calories
Apple	1	80
Banana	1	100
Beans, green cooked	½ cup	18
Bread, whole wheat	1 slice	56
Butter	1 tablespoon	100
Carrot	1 medium	34
Cheese	1 ounce	107–14
Corn on the cob	5½ inches	160
Egg	1 large	80
Ice cream	½ cup	135
Kidney beans, cooked	½ cup	110
Meat	3 ounces	200–250
Milk, skim	1 cup	85
Milk, whole	1 cup	150
Orange	1	65
Peach	1	38
Peanuts	1 ounce	172
Pear	1	100
Peas	½ cup	86
Potato chips	10 chips	115
Rice, cooked	½ cup	110
Shrimp	3 ounces	78
Tuna	3 ounces	78
Yogurt, low fat	1 cup	140

From K. N. Prasad and K. C. Prasad, *Fight Cancer with Vitamins and Supplements: A Guide to Prevention and Treatment*, Rochester, Vt.: Healing Arts Press, 2001.

TABLE A.23. FAT CONTENT
OF SELECTED FOODS

Food	Portion size	Grams/Portion
Avocado	⅛	4
Bacon, crisp	2 slices	6
Beef, roast	3 ounces	26
Biscuit	1	4
Bread, whole wheat	1 slice	1
Cheese, cheddar	1 ounce	9
Chicken, baked, with skin	3 ounces	11
Chicken, baked, without skin	3 ounces	6
Cornbread	1 piece	7
Egg, boiled	1	6
Ice cream	½ cup	7
Margarine	1 teaspoon	4
Mayonnaise	1 tablespoon	11
Milk, skim	1 cup	1
Milk, whole	1 cup	8
Oatmeal, cooked	½ cup	1
Peanut butter	1 tablespoon	7
Pork chop	3 ounces	19
Shrimp	3 ounces	0.9
Sour cream	1 tablespoon	3
Tuna	3 ounces	0.9
Vegetable oil	1 teaspoon	5
Yogurt, low fat	1 cup	4

From K. N. Prasad and K. C. Prasad, *Fight Cancer with Vitamins and Supplements: A Guide to Prevention and Treatment*, Rochester, Vt.: Healing Arts Press, 2001.

TABLE A.24. FIBER CONTENT
OF SELECTED FOODS

Food	Portion size	Grams/Portion
Apple, with skin	1	3
Bread, white	1 slice	0.8
Bread, whole wheat	1 slice	1.3
Broccoli	½ cup	3.2
Carrot, raw	1 medium	2.4
Cereal, all-bran	1 cup	25.6
Cereal, raisin bran	1 cup	6
Corn	½ cup	4.6
Muffin, bran	1	4.2
Pear, with skin	1	3.8
Raspberries	½ cup	4.6

From K. N. Prasad and K. C. Prasad, *Fight Cancer with Vitamins and Supplements: A Guide to Prevention and Treatment*, Rochester, Vt.: Healing Arts Press, 2001.

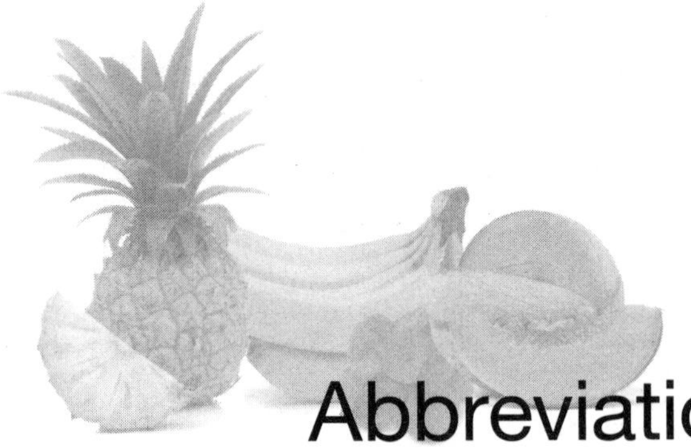

Abbreviations and Terminologies

3-NP: 3-Nitropropionic acid

3-NT: 3-Nitrotyrosine

4-HNE: 4-Hydroxynonenal

8-OHdG: 8-Hydroxy-2-deoxyguanosine

ARE: antioxidant response element

BDNF: brain-derived neurotrophic factor

CAG: cytosine, adenine and guanosine, a trinucleotide that codes for making glutamine

CB-1: cannabinoid receptor-1

COX: cyclooxygenase

CRP: C-reactive protein

CSF: cerebrospinal fluid

DA: dopamine

DBS: deep brain stimulation

EMF: electromagnetic field

EMP: electromagnetic pulse

GABA: gamma-aminobutyric acid

GDNF: glia cell–derived neurotrophic factor

GLT-1: glutamate transporter-1

GPX: glutathione peroxidase

H_2O_2: hydrogen peroxide

HO-1: heme oxygenase

IL-6: interleukin-6

MAO: monoamine oxidase

MCI: mild cognitive impairment

MDA: malondialdehyde

MPTP: 1-Methyl-4-phenyl 1,2,3,6-tetrahydropyridine

MRI: magnetic resonance imaging

NAC: N-acetylcysteine

NAD: nicotinamide adenine dinucleotide

NADH: reduced form of NAD

NFkappaB: nuclear factor kappa-beta

NGF: nerve growth factor

NMDA: N-methy-D-aspartate

NO: nitric oxide

Nrf2: nuclear factor-erythroid 2-related factor 2

NSAID: non-steroidal anti-inflammatory drug

PET: positron emission tomography

RBC: red blood cell

ROS: reactive oxygen species, also called free radicals

SN: substantia nigra

SOD: superoxide dismutase

TBARS: thiobarbituric acid reactive substances

TMS: transcranial magnetic stimulation

TNF-alpha: tumor necrosis factor-alpha

Bibliography

Abate, A., G. Yang, P. A. Dennery, et al. 2000. Synergistic inhibition of cyclo-oxygenase-2 expression by vitamin E and aspirin. *Free Radic Biol Med* 29, no. 11: 1135–42.

Albanes, D., O. P. Heinonen, J. K. Huttunen, et al. 1995. Effects of alpha-tocopherol and beta-carotene supplements on cancer incidence in the Alpha-Tocopherol Beta-Carotene Cancer Prevention Study. *Am J Clin Nutr* 62, no. 6 Suppl: 1427S–30S.

Alcain, F. J., and J. M. Villalba. 2009. Sirtuin inhibitors. *Expert Opin Ther Pat* 19, no. 3: 283–94.

Anderson, J. J. B., R. Martin, and S. C. Garner. 2005. *Nutrition and Health: An Introduction*. Durham, N.C.: Carolina Academic Press.

Andersen, J. K. 2004. Iron dysregulation and Parkinson's disease. *J Alzheimers Dis* 6, no. 6 Suppl: S47–52.

Andreassen, O. A., R. J. Ferrante, A. Dedeoglu, and M. F. Beal. 2001. Lipoic acid improves survival in transgenic mouse models of Huntington's disease. *Neuroreport* 12, no. 15: 3371–73.

Arduino, D. M., A. R. Esteves, S. M. Cardoso, and C. R. Oliveira. 2009. Endo-plasmic reticulum and mitochondria interplay mediates apoptotic cell death: relevance to Parkinson's disease. *Neurochem Int* 55, no. 5: 341–48.

Ariga, H., K. Takahashi-Niki, I. Kato, et al. 2013. Neuroprotective function of DJ-1 in Parkinson's disease. *Oxid Med Cell Longev* 2013: 683920.

Asmus, K-D., and M. Bonifacic, ed. 1994. "Free Radical Chemistry." In *Exercise and Oxygen Toxicity*. Edited by C. K. Pen, L. Packer, and O. Hänninen. New York: Elsevier.

Ballard, P. A., J. W. Tetrud, and J. W. Langston. 1985. Permanent human parkinsonism due to 1-methyl-4-phenyl-1,2,3,6-tetrahydropyridine (MPTP): seven cases. *Neurology* 35, no. 7: 949–56.

Bandopadhyay, R., A. E. Kingsbury, M. R. Cookson, et al. 2004. The expression of DJ-1 (PARK7) in normal human CNS and idiopathic Parkinson's disease. *Brain* 127 (Pt. 2): 420–30.

Banerjee, R., A. A. Starkov, M. F. Beal, and B. Thomas. 2009. Mitochondrial dysfunction in the limelight of Parkinson's disease pathogenesis. *Biochim Biophys Acta* 1792, no. 7: 651–63.

Barger, S. W., M. E. Goodwin, M. M. Porter, and M. L. Beggs. 2007. Glutamate release from activated microglia requires the oxidative burst and lipid peroxidation. *J Neurochem* 101, no. 5: 1205–13.

Batelli, S., D. Albani, R. Rametta, et al. 2008. DJ-1 modulates alpha-synuclein aggregation state in a cellular model of oxidative stress: relevance for Parkinson's disease and involvement of HSP70. *PLoS One* 3, no. 4: e1884.

Baum, M. K., A. Campa, S. Lai, et al. 2013. Effect of micronutrient supplementation on disease progression in asymptomatic, antiretroviral-naive, HIV-infected adults in Botswana: a randomized clinical trial. *JAMA* 310, no. 20: 2154–63.

Bergstrom, P., H. C. Andersson, Y. Gao, et al. 2011. Repeated transient sulforaphane stimulation in astrocytes leads to prolonged Nrf2-mediated gene expression and protection from superoxide-induced damage. *Neuropharmacology* 60, nos. 2–3: 343–53.

Bjorkblom, B., A. Adilbayeva, J. Maple-Grodem, et al. 2013. Parkinson's disease Protein DJ-1 Binds Metals and Protects against Metal-induced Cytotoxicity. *J Biol Chem* 288, no. 31: 22809–20.

Bjorkqvist, M., E. J. Wild, J. Thiele, et al. 2008. A novel pathogenic pathway of immune activation detectable before clinical onset in Huntington's disease. *J Exp Med* 205, no. 8: 1869–77.

Blandini, F., R. H. Porter, and J. T. Greenamyre. 1996. Glutamate and Parkinson's disease. *Mol Neurobiol* 12, no. 1: 73–94.

Blazquez, C., A. Chiarlone, O. Sagredo, et al. 2011. Loss of striatal type 1 cannabinoid receptors is a key pathogenic factor in Huntington's disease. *Brain* 134 (Pt. 1): 119–36.

Bolner, A., M. Pilleri, V. De Riva, and G. P. Nordera. 2011. Plasma and urinary HPLC-ED determination of the ratio of 8-OHdG/2-dG in Parkinson's disease. *Clin Lab* 57, nos. 11–12: 859–66.

Bonsi, P., D. Cuomo, B. Picconi, et al. 2007. Striatal metabotropic glutamate receptors as a target for pharmacotherapy in Parkinson's disease. *Amino Acids* 32, no. 2: 189–95.

Bouchard, J., J. Truong, K. Bouchard, et al. 2012. Cannabinoid receptor 2 signaling in peripheral immune cells modulates disease onset and severity in mouse models of Huntington's disease. *J Neurosci* 32, no. 50: 18259–68.

Brinjikji, W., A. A. Rabinstein, and H. J. Cloft. 2012. Hospitalization costs for acute ischemic stroke patients treated with intravenous thrombolysis in the United States are substantially higher than medicare payments. *Stroke* 43, no. 4: 1131–33.

Browne, S. E. 2008. Mitochondria and Huntington's disease pathogenesis: insight from genetic and chemical models. *Ann NY Acad Sci* 1147: 358–82.

Browne, S. E., A. C. Bowling, U. MacGarvey, et al. 1997. Oxidative damage and metabolic dysfunction in Huntington's disease: selective vulnerability of the basal ganglia. *Ann Neurol* 41, no. 5: 646–53.

Browne, S. E., and M. F. Beal. 2006. Oxidative damage in Huntington's disease pathogenesis. *Antioxid Redox Signal* 8, nos. 11–12: 2061–73.

Brusa, L., A. Orlacchio, V. Moschella, et al. 2009. Treatment of the symptoms of Huntington's disease: preliminary results comparing aripiprazole and tetrabenazine. *Mov Disord* 24, no. 1: 126–29.

Bueler, H. 2009. Impaired mitochondrial dynamics and function in the pathogenesis of Parkinson's disease. *Exp Neurol* 218, no. 2: 235–46.

Cadenas, E. P., and L. Packer. 1996. *Handbook of Antioxidants.* New York: Marcel Dekker, Inc.

Chae, S. W., B. Y. Kang, O. Hwang, and H. J. Choi. 2008. Cyclooxygenase-2 is involved in oxidative damage and alpha-synuclein accumulation in dopaminergic cells. *Neurosci Lett* 436, no. 2: 205–9.

Chan, K., X. D. Han, and Y. W. Kan. 2001. An important function of Nrf2 in combating oxidative stress: detoxification of acetaminophen. *Proc Natl Acad Sci USA* 98, no. 8: 4611–16.

Charvin, D., E. Roze, V. Perrin, et al. 2008. Haloperidol protects striatal neurons from dysfunction induced by mutated huntingtin in vivo. *Neurobiol Dis* 29, no. 1: 22–29.

Charvin, D., P. Vanhoutte, C. Pages, et al. 2005. Unraveling a role for dopamine in Huntington's disease: the dual role of reactive oxygen species and D2 receptor stimulation. *Proc Natl Acad Sci USA* 102, no. 34: 12218–23.

Chaturvedi, R. K., S. Shukla, K. Seth, et al. 2006. Neuroprotective and neuro-rescue effect of black tea extract in 6-hydroxydopamine-lesioned rat model of Parkinson's disease. *Neurobiol Dis* 22, no. 2: 421–34.

Chen, C. M., Y. R. Wu, M. L. Cheng, et al. 2007. Increased oxidative damage and mitochondrial abnormalities in the peripheral blood of Huntington's disease patients. *Biochem Biophys Res Commun* 359, no. 2: 335–40.

Chen, R. S., C. C. Huang, and N. S. Chu. 1997. Coenzyme Q10 treatment in mitochondrial encephalomyopathies. Short-term double-blind, crossover study. *Eur Neurol* 37, no. 4: 212–18.

Chinta, S. J., and J. K. Andersen. 2005. Dopaminergic neurons. *Int J Biochem Cell Biol* 37, no. 5: 942–46.

Choi, D. H., A. C. Cristovao, S. Guhathakurta, et al. 2012. NADPH oxidase 1-mediated oxidative stress leads to dopamine neuron death in Parkinson's disease. *Antioxid Redox Signal* 16, no. 10: 1033–45.

Choi, H. K., Y. R. Pokharel, S. C. Lim, et al. 2009. Inhibition of liver fibrosis by solubilized coenzyme Q10: Role of Nrf2 activation in inhibiting transforming growth factor-beta1 expression. *Toxicol Appl Pharmacol* 240, no. 3: 377–84.

Choi, J. Y., C. S. Park, D. J. Kim, et al. 2002. Prevention of nitric oxide-mediated 1-methyl-4-phenyl-1,2,3,6-tetrahydropyridine-induced Parkinson's disease in mice by tea phenolic epigallocatechin 3-gallate. *Neurotoxicology* 23, no. 3: 367–74.

Coelho, F. G., T. M. Vital, A. M. Stein, et al. 2014. Acute aerobic exercise increases brain-derived neurotrophic factor levels in elderly with Alzheimer's disease. *J Alzheimers Dis* 39, no. 2: 401–8.

Colin-Gonzalez, A. L., A. Luna-Lopez, M. Konigsberg, et al. 2014. Early modulation of the transcription factor Nrf2 in rodent striatal slices by quinolinic acid, a toxic metabolite of the kynurenine pathway. *Neuroscience* 260C: 130–39.

Colle, D., J. M. Hartwig, F. A. Soares, and M. Farina. 2012. Probucol modulates oxidative stress and excitotoxicity in Huntington's disease models in vitro. *Brain Res Bull* 87, nos. 4–5: 397–405.

Combs Jr., G. F. 1998. *The Vitamins: Fundamental Aspects in Nutrition and Health*, 2nd Edition. San Diego: Academic Press.

Cotran, R. S., V. Kumar, and T. Collins, ed. 1999. *Disease of Immunity, Pathologic Basis of Disease*. New York: W. B. Saunders Company.

Cui, L., H. Jeong, F. Borovecki, et al. 2006. Transcriptional repression of PGC-1alpha by mutant huntingtin leads to mitochondrial dysfunction and neurodegeneration. *Cell* 127, no. 1: 59–69.

da Costa, C. A. 2007. DJ-1: a newcomer in Parkinson's disease pathology. *Curr Mol Med* 7, no. 7: 650–57.

de Rijk, M. C., M. M. Breteler, J. H. den Breeijen, et al. 1997. Dietary antioxidants and Parkinson's disease. The Rotterdam Study. *Arch Neurol* 54, no. 6: 762–65.

de Yebenes, J. G., B. Landwehrmeyer, F. Squitieri, et al. 2011. Pridopidine for the treatment of motor function in patients with Huntington's disease (MermaiHD): a phase 3, randomised, double-blind, placebo-controlled trial. *Lancet Neurol* 10, no. 12: 1049–57.

Desplats, P., H. J. Lee, E. J. Bae, et al. 2009. Inclusion formation and neuronal cell death through neuron-to-neuron transmission of alpha-synuclein. *Proc Natl Acad Sci USA* 106, no. 31: 13010–15.

Devaraj, S., R. Tang, B. Adams-Huet, et al. 2007. Effect of high-dose alpha-tocopherol supplementation on biomarkers of oxidative stress and inflammation and carotid atherosclerosis in patients with coronary artery disease. *Am J Clin Nutr* 86, no. 5: 1392–98.

Devi, L., and H. K. Anandatheerthavarada. 2010. Mitochondrial trafficking of APP and alpha synuclein: Relevance to mitochondrial dysfunction in Alzheimer's and Parkinson's diseases. *Biochim Biophys Acta* 1802, no. 1: 11–19.

Dexter, D. T., A. E. Holley, W. D. Flitter, et al. 1994. Increased levels of lipid hydroperoxides in the parkinsonian substantia nigra: an HPLC and ESR study. *Mov Disord* 9, no. 1: 92–97.

Dodson, M. W., and M. Guo. 2007. PINK1, PARKIN, DJ-1 and mitochondrial dysfunction in Parkinson's disease. *Curr Opin Neurobiol* 17, no. 3: 331–37.

Domingues, A. F., D. M. Arduino, A. R. Esteves, et al. 2008. Mitochondria and ubiquitin-proteasomal system interplay: relevance to Parkinson's disease. *Free Radic Biol Med* 45, no. 6: 820–25.

Ebadi, M., and S. K. Sharma. 2003. Peroxynitrite and mitochondrial dysfunction in the pathogenesis of Parkinson's disease. *Antioxid Redox Signal* 5, no. 3: 319–35.

Ebadi, M., S. K. Srinivasan, and M. D. Baxi. 1996. Oxidative stress and antioxidant therapy in Parkinson's disease. *Prog Neurobiol* 48, no. 1: 1–19.

el-Agnaf, O. M., and G. B. Irvine. 2002. Aggregation and neurotoxicity of alpha-synuclein and related peptides. *Biochem Soc Trans* 30, no. 4: 559–65.

Enochs, W. S., T. Sarna, L. Zecca, et al. 1994. The roles of neuromelanin, binding of metal ions, and oxidative cytotoxicity in the pathogenesis of Parkinson's disease: a hypothesis. *J Neural Transm Park Dis Dement Sect* 7, no. 2: 83–100.

Erickson, J. T., T. A. Brosenitsch, and D. M. Katz. 2001. Brain-derived neuro-trophic factor and glial cell line-derived neurotrophic factor are required simultaneously for survival of dopaminergic primary sensory neurons in vivo. *J Neurosci* 21, no. 2: 581–89.

Esmaeilzadeh, M., L. Farde, P. Karlsson, et al. 2011. Extrastriatal dopamine D(2) receptor binding in Huntington's disease. *Hum Brain Mapp* 32, no. 10: 1626–36.

Esteves, A. R., D. M. Arduino, R. H. Swerdlow, et al. 2009. Oxidative Stress involvement in alpha-synuclein oligomerization in Parkinson's disease cybrids. *Antioxid Redox Signal* 11, no. 3: 439–48.

Etminan, M., S. S. Gill, and A. Samii. 2005. Intake of vitamin E, vitamin C, and carotenoids and the risk of Parkinson's disease: a meta-analysis. *Lancet Neurol* 4, no. 6: 362–65.

Fahn, S. 1992. A pilot trial of high-dose alpha-tocopherol and ascorbate in early Parkinson's disease. *Ann Neurol* 32 Suppl: S128–32.

———. 2005. Does levodopa slow or hasten the rate of progression of Parkin-son's disease? *J Neurol* 252 Suppl 4: IV37–IV42.

Fahn, S., D. Oakes, I. Shoulson, et al. 2004. Levodopa and the progression of Parkinson's disease. *N Engl J Med* 351, no. 24: 2498–508.

Fan, M. M., and L. A. Raymond. 2007. N-methyl-D-aspartate (NMDA) recep-tor function and excitotoxicity in Huntington's disease. *Prog Neurobiol* 81, nos. 5–6: 272–93.

Farina, N., M. G. Isaac, A. R. Clark, et al. 2012. Vitamin E for Alzheimer's dementia and mild cognitive impairment. *Cochrane Database Syst Rev* 11: CD002854.

Fernandez-Calle, P., F. J. Jimenez-Jimenez, J. A. Molina, et al. 1993. Serum lev-els of ascorbic acid (vitamin C) in patients with Parkinson's disease. *J Neu-rol Sci* 118, no. 1: 25–28.

Fessel, J. P., C. Hulette, S. Powell, et al. 2003. Isofurans, but not F2-isoprostanes, are increased in the substantia nigra of patients with Parkinson's disease and with dementia with Lewy body disease. *J Neurochem* 85, no. 3: 645–50.

Fitzgerald, J. C., and H. Plun-Favreau. 2008. Emerging pathways in genetic Par-kinson's disease: autosomal-recessive genes in Parkinson's disease—a com-mon pathway? *FEBS J* 275, no. 23: 5758–66.

Fitzmaurice, P. S., L. Ang, M. Guttman, et al. 2003. Nigral glutathione defi-ciency is not specific for idiopathic Parkinson's disease. *Mov Disord* 18, no. 9: 969–76.

Fleming, J. T., W. He, C. Hao, et al. 2013. The Purkinje neuron acts as a central regulator of spatially and functionally distinct cerebellar precursors. *Dev Cell* 27, no. 3: 278–92.

Forrest, C. M., G. M. Mackay, N. Stoy, et al. 2010. Blood levels of kynurenines, interleukin-23 and soluble human leucocyte antigen-G at different stages of Huntington's disease. *J Neurochem* 112, no. 1: 112–22.

Fox, J. H., J. A. Kama, G. Lieberman, et al. 2007. Mechanisms of copper ion mediated Huntington's disease progression. *PLoS ONE* 2, no. 3: e334.

Frei, B. 1994. *Natural Antioxidants in Human Health and Disease.* New York: Academic Press.

Fu, Y., S. Zheng, J. Lin, et al. 2008. Curcumin protects the rat liver from CCl4-caused injury and fibrogenesis by attenuating oxidative stress and suppressing inflammation. *Mol Pharmacol* 73, no. 2: 399–409.

Galvin, J. E. 2006. Interaction of alpha-synuclein and dopamine metabolites in the pathogenesis of Parkinson's disease: a case for the selective vulnerability of the substantia nigra. *Acta Neuropathol* 112, no. 2: 115–26.

Gan, L., M. R. Vargas, D. A. Johnson, and J. A. Johnson. 2012. Astrocyte-specific overexpression of Nrf2 delays motor pathology and synuclein aggregation throughout the CNS in the alpha-synuclein mutant (A53T) mouse model. *J Neurosci* 32, no. 49: 17775–87.

Gandhi, P. N., S. G. Chen, and A. L. Wilson-Delfosse. 2009. Leucine-rich repeat kinase 2 (LRRK2): a key player in the pathogenesis of Parkinson's disease. *J Neurosci Res* 87, no. 6: 1283–95.

Gandhi, S., M. M. Muqit, L. Stanyer, et al. 2006. PINK1 protein in normal human brain and Parkinson's disease. *Brain* 129 (Pt. 7): 1720–31.

Gan-Or, Z., L. J. Ozelius, A. Bar-Shira, et al. 2013. The p.L302P mutation in the lysosomal enzyme gene SMPD1 is a risk factor for Parkinson's disease. *Neurology* 80, no. 17: 1606–10.

Gao, H. M., P. T. Kotzbauer, K. Uryu, et al. 2008. Neuroinflammation and oxidation/nitration of alpha-synuclein linked to dopaminergic neurodegeneration. *J Neurosci* 28, no. 30: 7687–98.

Gao, L., J. Wang, K. R. Sekhar, et al. 2007. Novel n-3 fatty acid oxidation products activate Nrf2 by destabilizing the association between Keap1 and Cullin3. *J Biol Chem* 282, no. 4: 2529–37.

Garske, A. L., B. C. Smith, and J. M. Denu. 2007. Linking SIRT2 to Parkinson's disease. *ACS Chem Biol* 2, no. 8: 529–32.

Gautier, C. A., T. Kitada, and J. Shen. 2008. Loss of PINK1 causes mitochondrial functional defects and increased sensitivity to oxidative stress. *Proc Natl Acad Sci USA* 105, no. 32: 11364–69.

Gaziano, J. M., H. D. Sesso, W. G. Christen, et al. 2012. Multivitamins in the prevention of cancer in men: the Physicians' Health Study II randomized controlled trial. *JAMA* 308, no. 18: 1871–80.

Gegg, M. E., J. M. Cooper, A. H. Schapira, and J. W. Taanman. 2009. Silencing of PINK1 expression affects mitochondrial DNA and oxidative phosphorylation in dopaminergic cells. *PLoS One* 4, no. 3: e4756.

Giaime, E., C. Sunyach, C. Druon, et al. 2010. Loss of function of DJ-1 triggered by Parkinson's disease-associated mutation is due to proteolytic resistance to caspase-6. *Cell Death Differ* 17, no. 1: 158–69.

Giasson, B. I., and V. M. Van Deerlin. 2008. Mutations in LRRK2 as a cause of Parkinson's disease. *Neurosignals* 16, no. 1: 99–105.

Glass, M., A. van Dellen, C. Blakemore, et al. 2004. Delayed onset of Huntington's disease in mice in an enriched environment correlates with delayed loss of cannabinoid CB1 receptors. *Neuroscience* 123, no. 1: 207–12.

Glass, M., M. Dragunow, and R. L. Faull. 1997. Cannabinoid receptors in the human brain: a detailed anatomical and quantitative autoradiographic study in the fetal, neonatal and adult human brain. *Neuroscience* 77, no. 2: 299–318.

———. 2000. The pattern of neurodegeneration in Huntington's disease: a comparative study of cannabinoid, dopamine, adenosine and GABA(A) receptor alterations in the human basal ganglia in Huntington's disease. *Neuroscience* 97, no. 3: 505–19.

Golbe, L. I., T. M. Farrell, and P. H. Davis. 1988. Case-control study of early life dietary factors in Parkinson's disease. *Arch Neurol* 45, no. 12: 1350–53.

Goldman, S. M., P. J. Quinlan, G. W. Ross, et al. 2012. Solvent exposures and Parkinson's disease risk in twins. *Ann Neurol* 71, no. 6: 776–84.

Goswami, A., P. Dikshit, A. Mishra, et al. 2006. Oxidative stress promotes mutant huntingtin aggregation and mutant huntingtin-dependent cell death by mimicking proteasomal malfunction. *Biochem Biophys Res Commun* 342, no. 1: 184–90.

Graham, R. K., M. A. Pouladi, P. Joshi, et al. 2009. Differential susceptibility to excitotoxic stress in YAC128 mouse models of Huntington's disease between initiation and progression of disease. *J Neurosci* 29, no. 7: 2193–204.

Green, K. N., J. S. Steffan, H. Martinez-Coria, et al. 2008. Nicotinamide restores cognition in Alzheimer's disease transgenic mice via a mechanism involving sirtuin inhibition and selective reduction of Thr231-phosphotau. J Neurosci 28: 11500–11510.

Gu, L., T. Cui, C. Fan, et al. 2009. Involvement of ERK1/2 signaling pathway in DJ-1-induced neuroprotection against oxidative stress. *Biochem Biophys Res Commun* 383, no. 4: 469–74.

Guarente, L. 2007. Sirtuins in aging and disease. *Cold Spring Harb Symp Quant Biol* 72: 483–88.

Hancock, D. B., E. R. Martin, J. M. Stajich, et al. 2007. Smoking, caffeine, and nonsteroidal anti-inflammatory drugs in families with Parkinson's disease. *Arch Neurol* 64, no. 4: 576–80.

Hands, S., M. U. Sajjad, M. J. Newton, and A. Wyttenbach. 2011. In vitro and in vivo aggregation of a fragment of huntingtin protein directly causes free radical production. *J Biol Chem* 286, no. 52: 44512–20.

Harms, A. S., S. Cao, A. L. Rowse, et al. 2013. MHCII is required for alpha-synuclein-induced activation of microglia, CD4 T cell proliferation, and dopaminergic neurodegeneration. *J Neurosci* 33, no. 23: 9592–600.

Hathorn, T., A. Snyder-Keller, and A. Messer. 2011. Nicotinamide improves motor deficits and upregulates PGC-1alpha and BDNF gene expression in a mouse model of Huntington's disease. *Neurobiol Dis* 41, no. 1: 43–50.

Hayes, J. D., S. A. Chanas, C. J. Henderson, et al. 2000. The Nrf2 transcription factor contributes both to the basal expression of glutathione S-transferases in mouse liver and to their induction by the chemopreventive synthetic antioxidants, butylated hydroxyanisole and ethoxyquin. *Biochem Soc Trans* 28, no. 2: 33–41.

Heim, C., W. Kolasiewicz, T. Kurz, and K. H. Sontag. 2001. Behavioral alterations after unilateral 6-hydroxydopamine lesions of the striatum. Effect of alpha-tocopherol. *Pol J Pharmacol* 53, no. 5: 435–48.

Hermel, E., J. Gafni, S. S. Propp, et al. 2004. Specific caspase interactions and amplification are involved in selective neuronal vulnerability in Huntington's disease. *Cell Death Differ* 11, no. 4: 424–38.

Hickey, M. A., A. Kosmalska, J. Enayati, et al. 2008. Extensive early motor and non-motor behavioral deficits are followed by striatal neuronal loss in knock-in Huntington's disease mice. *Neuroscience* 157, no. 1: 280–95.

Hickey, M. A., C. Zhu, V. Medvedeva, et al. 2012. Improvement of neuropathology and transcriptional deficits in CAG 140 knock-in mice supports a beneficial effect of dietary curcumin in Huntington's disease. *Mol Neurodegener* 7: 12.

Hickey, M. A., C. Zhu, V. Medvedeva, et al. 2012. Evidence for behavioral benefits of early dietary supplementation with CoEnzymeQ10 in a slowly progressing mouse model of Huntington's disease. *Mol Cell Neurosci* 49, no. 2: 149–57.

Hine, C. M., and J. R. Mitchell. 2012. Nrf2 and the phase II response in acute stress resistance induced by dietary restriction. *J Clin Exp Pathol* S4, no. 4.

Hoepken, H. H., S. Gispert, M. Azizov, et al. 2008. Parkinson patient fibroblasts show increased alpha-synuclein expression. *Exp Neurol* 212, no. 2: 307–13.

Hoffner, G., S. Soues, and P. Djian. 2007. Aggregation of expanded huntingtin in the brains of patients with Huntington disease. *Prion* 1, no. 1: 26–31.

Holland, E. C., and H. E. Varmus. 1998. Basic fibroblast growth factor induces cell migration and proliferation after glia-specific gene transfer in mice. *Proc Natl Acad Sci USA* 95, no. 3: 1218–23.

Holtmeier, W., and D. Kabelitz. 2005. Gammadelta T cells link innate and adaptive immune responses. *Chem Immunol Allergy* 86: 151–83.

Hori, K., D. Hatfield, F. Maldarelli, et al. 1997. Selenium supplementation suppresses tumor necrosis factor alpha-induced human immunodeficiency virus type 1 replication in vitro. *AIDS Res Hum Retroviruses* 13, no. 15: 1325–32.

Houlgatte, R., M. Mallat, P. Brachet, and A. Prochiantz. 1989. Secretion of nerve growth factor in cultures of glial cells and neurons derived from different regions of the mouse brain. *J Neurosci Res* 24, no. 2: 143–52.

Huntington Disease Collaborative Research Group. 1993. A novel gene containing a trinucleotide repeat that is expanded and unstable on Huntington's disease chromosomes. *Cell* 72: 971–83.

Im, J. Y., K. W. Lee, J. M. Woo, et al. 2012. DJ-1 induces thioredoxin 1 expression through the Nrf2 pathway. *Hum Mol Genet* 21, no. 13: 3013–24.

Investigators, Huntington Study Group HART. 2013. A randomized, double-blind, placebo-controlled trial of pridopidine in Huntington disease. *Mov Disord* 28, no. 10: 1407–15.

Itoh, K., T. Chiba, S. Takahashi, et al. 1997. An Nrf2/small Maf heterodimer mediates the induction of phase II detoxifying enzyme genes through antioxidant response elements. *Biochem Biophys Res Commun* 236, no. 2: 313–22.

Izumi, Y. 2013. [Dopaminergic neuroprotection via Nrf2-ARE pathway activation: identification of an activator from green perilla leaves]. *Yakugaku Zasshi* 133, no. 9: 983–88.

Jesudason, E. P., J. G. Masilamoni, B. S. Ashok, et al. 2008. Inhibitory effects of short-term administration of DL-alpha-lipoic acid on oxidative vulnerability induced by Abeta amyloid fibrils (25–35) in mice. *Mol Cell Biochem* 311, nos. 1–2: 145–56.

Ji, L., R. Liu, X. D. Zhang, et al. 2010. N-acetylcysteine attenuates phosgene-induced acute lung injury via up-regulation of Nrf2 expression. *Inhal Toxicol* 22, no. 7: 535–42.

Jia, H., X. Li, H. Gao, et al. 2008. High doses of nicotinamide prevent oxidative mitochondrial dysfunction in a cellular model and improve motor deficit in a Drosophila model of Parkinson's disease. *J Neurosci Res* 86, no. 9: 2083–90.

Jia, H., Z. Liu, X. Li, et al. 2010. Synergistic anti-Parkinsonism activity of high doses of B vitamins in a chronic cellular model. *Neurobiol Aging* 31, no. 4: 636–46.

Jiang, H., Y. Ren, E. Y. Yuen, et al. 2012. Parkin controls dopamine utilization in human midbrain dopaminergic neurons derived from induced pluripotent stem cells. *Nat Commun* 3: 668.

Jin, Y. N., Y. V. Yu, S. Gundemir, et al. 2013. Impaired mitochondrial dynamics and Nrf2 signaling contribute to compromised responses to oxidative stress in striatal cells expressing full-length mutant huntingtin. *PLoS ONE* 8, no. 3: e57932.

Junn, E., K. W. Lee, B. S. Jeong, et al. 2009. Repression of alpha-synuclein expression and toxicity by microRNA-7. *Proc Natl Acad Sci USA* 106, no. 31: 13052–57.

Kahle, P. J., J. Waak, and T. Gasser. 2009. DJ-1 and prevention of oxidative stress in Parkinson's disease and other age-related disorders. *Free Radic Biol Med* 47, no. 10: 1354–61.

Kaidery, N. A., R. Banerjee, L. Yang, et al. 2013. Targeting Nrf2-mediated gene transcription by extremely potent synthetic triterpenoids attenuate dopaminergic neurotoxicity in the MPTP mouse model of Parkinson's disease. *Antioxid Redox Signal* 18, no. 2: 139–57.

Kalia, L. V., S. K. Kalia, P. J. McLean, et al. 2013. Alpha-synuclein oligomers and clinical implications for Parkinson's disease. *Ann Neurol* 73, no. 2: 155–69.

Kalonia, H., and A. Kumar. 2011. Suppressing inflammatory cascade by cyclo-oxygenase inhibitors attenuates quinolinic acid induced Huntington's disease-like alterations in rats. *Life Sci* 88, nos. 17–18: 784–91.

Kalonia, H., P. Kumar, and A. Kumar. 2011. Attenuation of proinflammatory cytokines and apoptotic process by verapamil and diltiazem against quinolinic acid induced Huntington like alterations in rats. *Brain Res* 1372: 115–26.

Kandel, E. R., J. H. Schwartz, and T. M. Jessel. 2000. *Principles of Neural Science*. New York: McGraw-Hill.

Kehrer, J. P. and C. V. Smith, ed. 1994. *Free radicals in biology: sources, reactives, and roles in the etiology of human diseases*. Edited by B. Frei, *Natural Antioxidants in Human Health and Disease*. New York: Academy Press, Inc.

Kehry, M. R., and P. D. Hodgkin. 1994. B-cell activation by helper T-cell membranes. *Crit Rev Immunol* 14, nos. 3–4: 221–38.

Khaldy, H., G. Escames, J. Leon, et al. 2000. Comparative effects of melatonin, L-deprenyl, Trolox and ascorbate in the suppression of hydroxyl radical formation during dopamine auto-oxidation in vitro. *J Pineal Res* 29, no. 2: 100–107.

Khaldy, H., G. Escames, J. Leon, et al. 2003. Synergistic effects of melatonin and deprenyl against MPTP-induced mitochondrial damage and DA depletion. *Neurobiol Aging* 24, no. 3: 491–500.

Khoshnan, A., and P. H. Patterson. 2011. The role of IkappaB kinase complex in the neurobiology of Huntington's disease. *Neurobiol Dis* 43, no. 2: 305–11.

Kim, C., and S. J. Lee. 2008. Controlling the mass action of alpha-synuclein in Parkinson's disease. *J Neurochem* 107, no. 2: 303–16.

Kim, J., J. P. Moody, C. K. Edgerly, et al. 2010. Mitochondrial loss, dysfunction and altered dynamics in Huntington's disease. *Hum Mol Genet* 19, no. 20: 3919–35.

Kim, S. J., Y. J. Park, I. Y. Hwang, et al. 2012. Nuclear translocation of DJ-1 during oxidative stress-induced neuronal cell death. *Free Radic Biol Med* 53, no. 4: 936–50.

Kish, S. J., C. Morito, and O. Hornykiewicz. 1985. Glutathione peroxidase activity in Parkinson's disease brain. *Neurosci Lett* 58, no. 3: 343–46.

Kitamura, Y., S. Watanabe, M. Taguchi, et al. 2011. Neuroprotective effect of a new DJ-1-binding compound against neurodegeneration in Parkinson's disease and stroke model rats. *Mol Neurodegener* 6, no. 1: 48.

Klein, C., and K. Lohmann-Hedrich. 2007. Impact of recent genetic findings in Parkinson's disease. *Curr Opin Neurol* 20, no. 4: 453–64.

Kode, A., S. Rajendrasozhan, S. Caito, et al. 2008. Resveratrol induces glutathione synthesis by activation of Nrf2 and protects against cigarette smoke-mediated oxidative stress in human lung epithelial cells. *Am J Physiol Lung Cell Mol Physiol* 294, no. 3: L478–88.

Kraft, A. D., L. S. Kaltenbach, D. C. Lo, and G. J. Harry. 2012. Activated microglia proliferate at neurites of mutant huntingtin-expressing neurons. *Neurobiol Aging* 33, no. 3: 621 e17–33.

Kuhlmann, M. K., and N. W. Levin. 2008. Potential Interplay between Nutrition and Inflammation in Dialysis Patients. *Contrib Nephrol* 161: 76–82.

Kuhn, A., D. R. Goldstein, A. Hodges, et al. 2007. Mutant huntingtin's effects on striatal gene expression in mice recapitulate changes observed in human Huntington's disease brain and do not differ with mutant huntingtin length or wild-type huntingtin dosage. *Hum Mol Genet* 16, no. 15: 1845–61.

Kumar, P., and A. Kumar. 2009. Effect of lycopene and epigallocatechin-3-gallate against 3-nitropropionic acid induced cognitive dysfunction and glutathione depletion in rat: a novel nitric oxide mechanism. *Food Chem Toxicol* 47, no. 10: 2522–30.

Kumar, P., S. S. Padi, P. S. Naidu, and A. Kumar. 2006. Effect of resveratrol on 3-nitropropionic acid-induced biochemical and behavioural changes: possible neuroprotective mechanisms. *Behav Pharmacol* 17, nos. 5–6: 485–92.

Langermans, J. A., W. L. Hazenbos, and R. van Furth. 1994. Antimicrobial functions of mononuclear phagocytes. *J Immunol Methods* 174, nos. 1–2: 185–94.

Lastres-Becker, I., A. Ulusoy, N. G. Innamorato, et al. 2012. Alpha-synuclein expression and Nrf2 deficiency cooperate to aggravate protein aggregation, neuronal death and inflammation in early-stage Parkinson's disease. *Hum Mol Genet* 21, no. 14: 3173–92.

Lee, H. S., K. K. Jung, J. Y. Cho, et al. 2007. Neuroprotective effect of curcumin is mainly mediated by blockade of microglial cell activation. *Pharmazie* 62, no. 12: 937–42.

Lee, S. J. 2003. Alpha-synuclein aggregation: a link between mitochondrial defects and Parkinson's disease? *Antioxid Redox Signal* 5, no. 3: 337–48.

Lee, T. M., M. L. Wong, B. W. Lau, et al. 2014. Aerobic exercise interacts with neurotrophic factors to predict cognitive functioning in adolescents. *Psychoneuroendocrinology* 39: 214–24.

Lev, N., D. Ickowicz, Y. Barhum, et al. 2009. DJ-1 protects against dopamine toxicity. *J Neural Transm* 116, no. 2: 151–60.

Lev, N., Y. Barhum, N. S. Pilosof, et al. 2013. DJ-1 protects against dopamine toxicity: implications for Parkinson's disease and aging. *J Gerontol A Biol Sci Med Sci* 68, no. 3: 215–25.

Li, X. H., C. Y. Li, J. M. Lu, et al. 2012. Allicin ameliorates cognitive deficits ageing-induced learning and memory deficits through enhancing of Nrf2 antioxidant signaling pathways. *Neurosci Lett* 514, no. 1: 46–50.

Li, Y., W. Liu, T. F. Oo, et al. 2009. Mutant LRRK2(R1441G) BAC transgenic mice recapitulate cardinal features of Parkinson's disease. *Nat Neurosci* 12, no. 7: 826–28.

Litman, G. W., J. P. Cannon, and L. J. Dishaw. 2005. Reconstructing immune phylogeny: new perspectives. *Nat Rev Immunol* 5, no. 11: 866–79.

Liu, D., M. Pitta, and M. P. Mattson. 2008. Preventing NAD(+) depletion protects neurons against excitotoxicity: bioenergetic effects of mild mitochondrial uncoupling and caloric restriction. *Ann N Y Acad Sci* 1147: 275–82.

Liu, W., C. Vives-Bauza, R. Acin-Perez, et al. 2009. PINK1 defect causes mitochondrial dysfunction, proteasomal deficit and alpha-synuclein aggregation in cell-culture models of Parkinson's disease. *PLoS One* 4, no. 2: e4597.

Lou, H., X. Jing, X. Wei, et al. 2013. Naringenin protects against 6-OHDA-induced neurotoxicity via activation of the Nrf2/ARE signaling pathway. *Neuropharmacology* 79C: 380–88.

Ma, L., T. T. Cao, G. Kandpal, et al. 2010. Genome-wide microarray analysis of the differential neuroprotective effects of antioxidants in neuroblastoma cells overexpressing the familial Parkinson's disease alpha-synuclein A53T mutation. *Neurochem Res* 35, no. 1: 130–42.

MacDonald, M. E., C. M. Ambrose, M. P. Duyao, et al. 1993. A novel gene containing a trinucleotide repeat that is expanded and unstable on Huntington's disease chromosome. *Cell* 72: 971–83.

Mahdy, H. M., M. G. Tadros, M. R. Mohamed, et al. 2011. The effect of Ginkgo biloba extract on 3-nitropropionic acid-induced neurotoxicity in rats. *Neurochem Int* 59, no. 6: 770–78.

Maldonado, P. D., E. Molina-Jijon, J. Villeda-Hernandez, et al. 2010. NAD(P) H oxidase contributes to neurotoxicity in an excitotoxic/prooxidant model of Huntington's disease in rats: protective role of apocynin. *J Neurosci Res* 88, no. 3: 620–29.

Mandel, S., E. Grunblatt, P. Riederer, et al. 2003. Neuroprotective strategies in Parkinson's disease: an update on progress. *CNS Drugs* 17, no. 10: 729–62.

Marongiu, R., B. Spencer, L. Crews, et al. 2009. Mutant PINK1 induces mitochondrial dysfunction in a neuronal cell model of Parkinson's disease by disturbing calcium flux. *J Neurochem* 108, no. 6: 1561–74.

Martin, E., S. Betuing, C. Pages, et al. 2011. Mitogen- and stress-activated protein kinase 1-induced neuroprotection in Huntington's disease: role on chromatin remodeling at the PGC-1-alpha promoter. *Hum Mol Genet* 20, no. 12: 2422–34.

Martin, P., and S. J. Leibovich. 2005. Inflammatory cells during wound repair: the good, the bad and the ugly. *Trends Cell Biol* 15, no. 11: 599–607.

Martire, A., G. Calamandrei, F. Felici, et al. 2007. Opposite effects of the A2A receptor agonist CGS21680 in the striatum of Huntington's disease versus wild-type mice. *Neurosci Lett* 417, no. 1: 78–83.

Matzinger, P. 2002. The danger model: a renewed sense of self. *Science* 296, no. 5566: 301–5.

McGeer, P. L., and E. G. McGeer. 2008. Glial reactions in Parkinson's disease. *Mov Disord* 23, no. 4: 474–83.

Medzhitov, R. 2007. Recognition of microorganisms and activation of the immune response. *Nature* 449, no. 7164: 819–26.

Melamed, E., D. Offen, A. Shirvan, et al. 1998. Levodopa toxicity and apoptosis. *Ann Neurol* 44, no. 3, Suppl 1: S149–54.

Mena, I., K. Horiuchi, K. Burke, and G. C. Cotzias. 1969. Chronic manganese poisoning. Individual susceptibility and absorption of iron. *Neurology* 19, no. 10: 1000–6.

Meredith, G. E., S. Totterdell, M. Beales, and C. K. Meshul. 2009. Impaired glutamate homeostasis and programmed cell death in a chronic MPTP mouse model of Parkinson's disease. *Exp Neurol* 219, no. 1: 334–40.

Mievis, S., D. Blum, and C. Ledent. 2011. A2A receptor knockout worsens survival and motor behaviour in a transgenic mouse model of Huntington's disease. *Neurobiol Dis* 41, no. 2: 570–76.

Miller, B. R., J. L. Dorner, K. D. Bunner, et al. 2012. Up-regulation of GLT1 reverses the deficit in cortically evoked striatal ascorbate efflux in the R6/2 mouse model of Huntington's disease. *J Neurochem* 121, no. 4: 629–38.

Mitsui, T., Y. Kuroda, and R. Kaji. 2008. [Parkin and mitochondria]. *Brain Nerve* 60, no. 8: 923–29.

Niture, S. K., J. W. Kaspar, J. Shen, and A. K. Jaiswal. 2010. Nrf2 signaling and cell survival. *Toxicol Appl Pharmacol* 244, no. 1: 37–42.

Nunome, K., S. Miyazaki, M. Nakano, et al. 2008. Pyrroloquinoline quinone prevents oxidative stress-induced neuronal death probably through changes in oxidative status of DJ-1. *Biol Pharm Bull* 31, no. 7: 1321–26.

Olanow, C. W., and G. W. Arendash. 1994. Metals and free radicals in neurodegeneration. *Curr Opin Neurol* 7, no. 6: 548–58.

Ono, K., and M. Yamada. 2007. Vitamin A potently destabilizes preformed alpha-synuclein fibrils in vitro: implications for Lewy body diseases. *Neurobiol Dis* 25, no. 2: 446–54.

Ortiz, A. N., B. J. Kurth, G. L. Osterhaus, and M. A. Johnson. 2011. Impaired dopamine release and uptake in R6/1 Huntington's disease model mice. *Neurosci Lett* 492, no. 1: 11–14.

Ortiz, A. N., G. L. Osterhaus, K. Lauderdale, et al. 2012. Motor function and dopamine release measurements in transgenic Huntington's disease model rats. *Brain Res* 1450: 148–56.

Ortiz, G. G., F. P. Pacheco-Moises, V. M. Gomez-Rodriguez, et al. 2013. Fish oil, melatonin and vitamin E attenuates midbrain cyclooxygenase-2 activity and oxidative stress after administration of 1-methyl-4-phenyl-1,2,3,6-tetrahydropyridine. *Metab Brain Dis* 28, no. 4: 705–9.

Packer, L., M. Hiramatsu, and T. Yoshikawa. 1999. *Antioxidants Food Supplements in Human Health*. New York: Academic Press.

Paraskevas, G. P., E. Kapaki, O. Petropoulou, et al. 2003. Plasma levels of antioxidant vitamins C and E are decreased in vascular parkinsonism. *J Neurol Sci* 215, nos. 1–2: 51–55.

Parent, A., and M. B. Carpenter. 1995. *Carpenter's Human Anatomy*. Philadelphia: Williams and Wilkins.

Parihar, M. S., A. Parihar, M. Fujita, et al. 2009. Alpha-synuclein overexpression and aggregation exacerbates impairment of mitochondrial functions by augmenting oxidative stress in human neuroblastoma cells. *Int J Biochem Cell Biol* 41, no. 10: 2015–24.

Park, E. S., S. Y. Kim, J. I. Na, et al. 2007. Glutathione prevented dopamine-induced apoptosis of melanocytes and its signaling. *J Dermatol Sci* 47, no. 2: 141–49.

Parkinson's Study Group. 1993. Effects of tocopherol and deprenyl on the progression of disability in early parkinson's disease. *N Engl J Med* 328, no. 3:176–83.

Pasbakhsh, P., N. Omidi, K. Mehrannia, et al. 2008. The protective effect of vitamin E on locus coeruleus in early model of Parkinson's disease in rat: immunoreactivity evidence. *Iran Biomed J* 12, no. 4: 217–22.

Pavese, N., A. Gerhard, Y. F. Tai, et al. 2006. Microglial activation correlates with severity in Huntington disease: a clinical and PET study. *Neurology* 66, no. 11: 1638–43.

Pavese, N., M. Politis, Y. F. Tai, et al. 2010. Cortical dopamine dysfunction in symptomatic and premanifest Huntington's disease gene carriers. *Neurobiol Dis* 37, no. 2: 356–61.

Peairs, A. T., and J. W. Rankin. 2008. Inflammatory response to a high-fat, low-carbohydrate weight loss diet: effect of antioxidants. *Obesity* (Silver Spring) 16, no 7: 1573–78.

Peng, J., F. F. Stevenson, M. L. Oo, and J. K. Andersen. 2009. Iron-enhanced para-quat-mediated dopaminergic cell death due to increased oxidative stress as a consequence of microglial activation. *Free Radic Biol Med* 46, no. 2: 312–20.

Penugonda, S., S. Mare, G. Goldstein, et al. 2005. Effects of N-acetylcysteine amide (NACA), a novel thiol antioxidant against glutamate-induced cyto-toxicity in neuronal cell line PC12. *Brain Res* 1056, no. 2: 132–38.

Perez-De La Cruz, V., C. Gonzalez-Cortes, S. Galvan-Arzate, et al. 2005. Exci-totoxic brain damage involves early peroxynitrite formation in a model of Huntington's disease in rats: protective role of iron porphyrinate 5,10,15,20-tetrakis (4-sulfonatophenyl) porphyrinate iron (III). *Neurosci-ence* 135, no. 2: 463–74.

Peyser, C. E., M. Folstein, G. A. Chase, et al. 1995. Trial of d-alpha-tocopherol in Huntington's disease. *Am J Psychiatry* 152, no. 12: 1771–75.

Pezzoli, G., and E. Cereda. 2013. Exposure to pesticides or solvents and risk of Parkinson's disease. *Neurology* 80, no. 22: 2035–41.

Pintor, A., M. T. Tebano, A. Martire, et al. 2006. The cannabinoid receptor agonist WIN 55,212-2 attenuates the effects induced by quinolinic acid in the rat striatum. *Neuropharmacology* 51, no. 5: 1004–12.

Politis, M., N. Pavese, Y. F. Tai, et al. 2011. Microglial activation in regions related to cognitive function predicts disease onset in Huntington's disease: a multimodal imaging study. *Hum Brain Mapp* 32, no. 2: 258–70.

Powers, K. M., D. M. Kay, S. A. Factor, et al. 2008. Combined effects of smok-ing, coffee, and NSAIDs on Parkinson's disease risk. *Mov Disord* 23, no. 1: 88–95.

Prabhakaran, K., D. Ghosh, G. D. Chapman, and P. G. Gunasekar. 2008. Molecular mechanism of manganese exposure-induced dopaminergic toxic-ity. *Brain Res Bull* 76, no. 4: 361–67.

Prasad, J. E., B. Kumar, C. Andreatta, et al. 2004. Overexpression of alpha-synuclein decreased viability and enhanced sensitivity to prostaglandin E(2), hydrogen peroxide, and a nitric oxide donor in differentiated neuro-blastoma cells. *J Neurosci Res* 76, no. 3: 415–22.

Prasad, K. N. 2011. *Micronutrients in Health and Disease*. Boca Raton, Fla.: CRC Press.

Prasad, K. N., W. C. Cole, and K. C. Prasad. 2002. Risk factors for Alzheimer's disease: role of multiple antioxidants, non-steroidal anti-inflammatory and cholinergic agents alone or in combination in prevention and treatment. *J Am Coll Nutr* 21, no. 6: 506–22.

Prasad, K. N., A. R. Hovland, F. G. La Rosa, and P. G. Hovland. 1998. Prostaglandins as putative neurotoxins in Alzheimer's disease. *Proc Soc Exp Biol Med* 219, no. 2: 120–25.

Prasad, K. N., and R. Kumar. 1996. Effect of individual and multiple antioxidant vitamins on growth and morphology of human nontumorigenic and tumorigenic parotid acinar cells in culture. *Nutr Cancer* 26, no. 1: 11–19.

Prasad, K. N., B. Kumar, X. D. Yan, A. J. Hanson, and W. C. Cole. 2003. Alpha-tocopheryl succinate, the most effective form of vitamin E for adjuvant cancer treatment: a review. *J Am Coll Nutr* 22, no. 2: 108–17.

Prasad, K. N., F. G. La Rosa, and J. E. Prasad. 1998. Prostaglandins act as neurotoxin for differentiated neuroblastoma cells in culture and increase levels of ubiquitin and beta-amyloid. *In Vitro Cell Dev Biol Anim* 34, no. 3: 265–74.

Pringsheim, T., K. Wiltshire, L. Day, et al. 2012. The incidence and prevalence of Huntington's disease: a systematic review and meta-analysis. *Mov Disord* 27, no. 9: 1083–91.

Pryor, W. A., ed. 1994. *Oxidants and antioxidants*. Edited by B. Frei, *Natural Antioxidants in Human Health and Disease*. New York: Academy Press, Inc.

Racette, B. A., M. Aschner, T. R. Guilarte, et al. 2012. Pathophysiology of manganese-associated neurotoxicity. *Neurotoxicology* 33, no. 4: 881–86.

Rahman, S., K. Bhatia, A. Q. Khan, et al. 2008. Topically applied vitamin E prevents massive cutaneous inflammatory and oxidative stress responses induced by double application of 12-O-tetradecanoylphorbol-13-acetate (TPA) in mice. *Chem Biol Interact* 172, no. 3: 195–205.

Ramsey, C. P., C. A. Glass, M. B. Montgomery, et al. 2007. Expression of Nrf2 in neurodegenerative diseases. *J Neuropathol Exp Neurol* 66, no. 1: 75–85.

Rebec, G. V., S. J. Barton, A. M. Marseilles, and K. Collins. 2003. Ascorbate treatment attenuates the Huntington behavioral phenotype in mice. *Neuroreport* 14, no. 9: 1263–65.

Rebec, G. V., S. K. Conroy, and S. J. Barton. 2006. Hyperactive striatal neurons in symptomatic Huntington R6/2 mice: variations with behavioral state and repeated ascorbate treatment. *Neuroscience* 137, no. 1: 327–36.

Reynolds, A. D., J. G. Glanzer, I. Kadiu, et al. 2008. Nitrated alpha-synuclein-activated microglial profiling for Parkinson's disease. *J Neurochem* 104, no. 6: 1504–25.

Rivera-Mancia, S., I. Perez-Neri, C. Rios, et al. 2010. The transition metals copper and iron in neurodegenerative diseases. *Chem Biol Interact* 186, no. 2: 184–99.

Robinson, P., M. Lebel, and M. Cyr. 2008. Dopamine D1 receptor-mediated aggregation of N-terminal fragments of mutant huntingtin and cell death in a neuroblastoma cell line. *Neuroscience* 153, no. 3: 762–72.

Rogers, J., L-F. Lue, L. Brachova, et al. 1995. Inflammation as a response and a cause of Alzheimer's pathophysiology. *Dementia* 9: 133–38.

Rojas, P., P. Montes, C. Rojas, et al. 2012. Effect of a phytopharmaceutical medicine, Ginkgo biloba extract 761, in an animal model of Parkinson's disease: therapeutic perspectives. *Nutrition* 28, nos. 11–12: 1081–88.

Ruiz, C., M. J. Casarejos, A. Gomez, et al. 2012. Protection by glia-conditioned medium in a cell model of Huntington disease. *PLoS Curr* 4: e4fbca54a2028b.

Rus, H., C. Cudrici, and F. Niculescu. 2005. The role of the complement system in innate immunity. *Immunol Res* 33, no. 2: 103–12.

Ryter, A. 1985. Relationship between ultrastructure and specific functions of macrophages. *Comp Immunol Microbiol Infect Dis* 8, no. 2: 119–33.

Sadri-Vakili, G., and J. H. Cha. 2006. Histone deacetylase inhibitors: a novel therapeutic approach to Huntington's disease (complex mechanism of neuronal death). *Curr Alzheimer Res* 3, no. 4: 403–8.

———. 2006. Mechanisms of disease: histone modifications in Huntington's disease. *Nat Clin Pract Neurol* 2, no. 6: 330–38.

Sagredo, O., S. Gonzalez, I. Aroyo, et al. 2009. Cannabinoid CB2 receptor agonists protect the striatum against malonate toxicity: relevance for Huntington's disease. *Glia* 57, no. 11: 1154–67.

Salazar, J., N. Mena, S. Hunot, et al. 2008. Divalent metal transporter 1 (DMT1) contributes to neurodegeneration in animal models of Parkinson's disease. *Proc Natl Acad Sci USA* 105, no. 47: 18578–83.

Samii, A., M. Etminan, M. O. Wiens, and S. Jafari. 2009. NSAID use and the risk of Parkinson's disease: systematic review and meta-analysis of observational studies. *Drugs Aging* 26, no. 9: 769–79.

Sanchez Mejia, R. O., and R. M. Friedlander. 2001. Caspases in Huntington's disease. *Neuroscientist* 7, no. 6: 480–89.

Sandhir, R., A. Sood, A. Mehrotra, and S. S. Kamboj. 2012. N-Acetylcysteine reverses mitochondrial dysfunctions and behavioral abnormalities in 3-nitropropionic acid-induced Huntington's disease. *Neurodegener Dis* 9, no. 3: 145–57.

Sandhu, J. K., S. Pandey, M. Ribecco-Lutkiewicz, et al. 2003. Molecular mechanisms of glutamate neurotoxicity in mixed cultures of NT2-derived neurons and astrocytes: protective effects of coenzyme Q10. *J Neurosci Res* 72, no. 6: 691–703.

Sano, M., C. Ernesto, R. G. Thomas, et al. 1997. A controlled trial of selegiline, alpha-tocopherol, or both as treatment for Alzheimer's disease. The Alzheimer's Disease Cooperative Study. *N Engl J Med* 336, no. 17: 1216–22.

Sanyal, J., S. K. Bandyopadhyay, T. K. Banerjee, et al. 2009. Plasma levels of lipid peroxides in patients with Parkinson's disease. *Eur Rev Med Pharmacol Sci* 13, no. 2: 129–32.

Saw, C. L., A. Y. Yang, Y. Guo, and A. N. Kong. 2013. Astaxanthin and omega-3 fatty acids individually and in combination protect against oxidative stress via the Nrf2-ARE pathway. *Food Chem Toxicol* 62: 869–75.

Sawada, M., K. Imamura, and T. Nagatsu. 2006. Role of cytokines in inflammatory process in Parkinson's disease. *J Neural Transm Suppl* 70: 373–81.

Schipper, H. M., A. Liberman, and E. G. Stopa. 1998. Neural heme oxygenase-1 expression in idiopathic Parkinson's disease. *Exp Neurol* 150, no. 1: 60–68.

Schubert, D., H. Kimura, and P. Maher. 1992. Growth factors and vitamin E modify neuronal glutamate toxicity. *Proc Natl Acad Sci USA* 89, no. 17: 8264–67.

Sen, C. K., L. Packer, and P. A. Baeuerle. 1999. *Antioxidants and Redox Regulation of Genes*. New York: Academic Press.

Shalit, F., B. Sredni, L. Stern, et al. 1994. Elevated interleukin-6 secretion levels by mononuclear cells of Alzheimer's patients. *Neurosci Lett* 174, no. 2: 130–32.

Shils, M. E., M. Shike, A. C. Ross, et al. 2005. *Modern Nutrition in Health and Disease*, 10th Edition. Philadelphia: Lippincott Williams and Wilkins.

Shoulson, I. 1998. DATATOP: a decade of neuroprotective inquiry. Parkinson Study Group. Deprenyl And Tocopherol Antioxidative Therapy Of Parkinsonism. *Ann Neurol* 44, no. 3 Suppl 1: S160–66.

Shults, C. W., D. Oakes, K. Kieburtz, et al. 2002. Effects of coenzyme Q10 in early Parkinson's disease: evidence of slowing of the functional decline. *Arch Neurol* 59, no. 10: 1541–50.

Silva-Adaya, D., V. Perez-De La Cruz, M. N. Herrera-Mundo, et al. 2008. Excitotoxic damage, disrupted energy metabolism, and oxidative stress in the rat brain: antioxidant and neuroprotective effects of L-carnitine. *J Neurochem* 105, no. 3: 677–89.

Smith, K. M., S. Matson, W. R. Matson, et al. 2006. Dose ranging and efficacy study of high-dose coenzyme Q10 formulations in Huntington's disease mice. *Biochim Biophys Acta* 1762, no. 6: 616–26.

Smith, M. A., L. M. Sayre, V. M. Monnier, and G. Perry. 1995. Radical AGEing in Alzheimer's disease. *Trends Neurosci* 18, no. 4: 172–76.

Sofic, E., A. Sapcanin, I. Tahirovic, et al. 2006. Antioxidant capacity in post-mortem brain tissues of Parkinson's and Alzheimer's diseases. *J Neural Transm Suppl* 71: 39–43.

Sproul, T. W., P. C. Cheng, M. L. Dykstra, and S. K. Pierce. 2000. A role for MHC class II antigen processing in B cell development. *Int Rev Immunol* 19, no. 2–3: 139–55.

Steele, M. L., S. Fuller, M. Patel, et al. 2013. Effect of Nrf2 activators on release of glutathione, cysteinylglycine and homocysteine by human U373 astroglial cells. *Redox Biol* 1, no. 1: 441–45.

Storch, A., W. H. Jost, P. Vieregge, et al. 2007. Randomized, double-blind, placebo-controlled trial on symptomatic effects of coenzyme Q(10) in Parkinson's disease. *Arch Neurol* 64, no. 7: 938–44.

Su, B., H. Liu, X. Wang, et al. 2009. Ectopic localization of FOXO3a protein in Lewy bodies in Lewy body dementia and Parkinson's disease. *Mol Neurodegener* 4: 32.

Suh, J. H., S. V. Shenvi, B. M. Dixon, et al. 2004. Decline in transcriptional activity of Nrf2 causes age-related loss of glutathione synthesis, which is reversible with lipoic acid. *Proc Natl Acad Sci USA* 101, no. 10: 3381–86.

Suzuki, Y. J., B. B. Aggarwal, and L. Packer. 1992. Alpha-lipoic acid is a potent inhibitor of NF-kappa B activation in human T cells. *Biochem Biophys Res Commun* 189, no. 3: 1709–15.

Tai, Y. F., N. Pavese, A. Gerhard, et al. 2007. Microglial activation in presymptomatic Huntington's disease gene carriers. *Brain* 130, Pt. 7: 1759–66.

Tamminga, C., T. Hashimoto, D. W. Volk, and D. A. Lewis. 2004. GABA neurons in the human prefrontal cortex. *Am J Psychiatry* 161, no. 10: 1764.

Tanner, C. M., S. M. Goldman, D. A. Aston, et al. 2002. Smoking and Parkinson's disease in twins. *Neurology* 58, no. 4: 581–88.

Tasset, I., A. J. Pontes, A. J. Hinojosa, et al. 2011. Olive oil reduces oxidative damage in a 3-nitropropionic acid-induced Huntington's disease-like rat model. *Nutr Neurosci* 14, no. 3: 106–11.

Tasset, I., A. Perez-Herrera, F. J. Medina, et al. 2013. Extremely low-frequency electromagnetic fields activate the antioxidant pathway Nrf2 in a Huntington's disease-like rat model. *Brain Stimul* 6, no. 1: 84–86.

Thomas, E. A., G. Coppola, P. A. Desplats, et al. 2008. The HDAC inhibitor 4b ameliorates the disease phenotype and transcriptional abnormalities in Huntington's disease transgenic mice. *Proc Natl Acad Sci USA* 105, no. 40: 15564–69.

Thomas, K. J., M. K. McCoy, J. Blackinton, et al. 2011. DJ-1 acts in parallel to the PINK1/PARKIN pathway to control mitochondrial function and autophagy. *Hum Mol Genet* 20, no. 1: 40–50.

Thompson, R. F. 2000. *The Brain: An Introduction to Neuroscience.* New York: Worth Publishers.

Toro, R., M. Perron, B. Pike, et al. 2008. Brain size and folding of the human cerebral cortex. *Cereb Cortex* 18, no. 10: 2352–57.

Trujillo, J., Y. I. Chirino, E. Molina-Jijon, et al. 2013. Renoprotective effect of the antioxidant curcumin: recent findings. *Redox Biol* 1, no. 1: 448–56.

Tsunemi, T., T. D. Ashe, B. E. Morrison, et al. 2012. PGC-1alpha rescues Huntington's disease proteotoxicity by preventing oxidative stress and promoting TFEB function. *Sci Transl Med* 4, no. 142: 142ra97.

Tunez, I., and A. Santamaria. 2009. [Model of Huntington's disease induced with 3-nitropropionic acid]. *Rev Neurol* 48, no. 8: 430–34.

Vaillancourt, F., H. Fahmi, Q. Shi, et al. 2008. 4-Hydroxynonenal induces apoptosis in human osteoarthritic chondrocytes: the protective role of glutathione-S-transferase. *Arthritis Res Ther* 10, no. 5: R107.

Vamos, E., K. Voros, L. Vecsei, and P. Klivenyi. 2010. Neuroprotective effects of L-carnitine in a transgenic animal model of Huntington's disease. *Biomed Pharmacother* 64, no. 4: 282–86.

Van Den Eeden, S. K., C. M. Tanner, A. L. Bernstein, et al. 2003. Incidence of Parkinson's disease: variation by age, gender, and race/ethnicity. *Am J Epidemiol* 157, no. 11: 1015–22.

van der Mark, M., M. Brouwer, H. Kromhout, et al. 2012. Is pesticide use related to Parkinson's disease? Some clues to heterogeneity in study results. *Environ Health Perspect* 120, no. 3: 340–47.

Van Laere, K., C. Casteels, I. Dhollander, et al. 2010. Widespread decrease of type 1 cannabinoid receptor availability in Huntington disease in vivo. *J Nucl Med* 51, no. 9: 1413–17.

Varghese, M., M. Pandey, A. Samanta, et al. 2009. Reduced NADH coenzyme Q dehydrogenase activity in platelets of Parkinson's disease, but not Parkinson plus patients, from an Indian population. *J Neurol Sci* 279, no. 1–2: 39–42.

Verbeek, M. M., I. Otte-Holler, J. R. Westphal, et al. 1994. Accumulation of intercellular adhesion molecule-1 in senile plaques in brain tissue of patients with Alzheimer's disease. *Am J Pathol* 144, no. 1: 104–16.

Virmani, A., F. Gaetani, and Z. Binienda. 2005. Effects of metabolic modifiers such as carnitines, coenzyme Q10, and PUFAs against different forms of neurotoxic insults: metabolic inhibitors, MPTP, and methamphetamine. *Ann NY Acad Sci* 1053: 183–91.

Wang, X., A. Sirianni, Z. Pei, et al. 2011. The melatonin MT1 receptor axis modulates mutant Huntingtin-mediated toxicity. *J Neurosci* 31, no. 41: 14496–507.

Weber, C. A., and M. E. Ernst. 2006. Antioxidants, supplements, and Parkinson's disease. *Ann Pharmacother* 40, no. 5: 935–38.

Williams, R. W., and K. Herrup. 1988. The control of neuron number. *Annu Rev Neurosci* 11: 423–53.

Willison, L. D., T. Kudo, D. H. Loh, et al. 2013. Circadian dysfunction may be a key component of the non-motor symptoms of Parkinson's disease: insights from a transgenic mouse model. *Exp Neurol* 243: 57–66.

Wilms, H., L. Zecca, P. Rosenstiel, et al. 2007. Inflammation in Parkinson's diseases and other neurodegenerative diseases: cause and therapeutic implications. *Curr Pharm Des* 13, no. 18: 1925–28.

Wood, L. G., M. L. Garg, H. Powell, and P. G. Gibson. 2008. Lycopene-rich treatments modify noneosinophilic airway inflammation in asthma: proof of concept. *Free Radic Res* 42, no. 1: 94–102.

Wruck, C. J., M. E. Gotz, T. Herdegen, et al. 2008. Kavalactones protect neural cells against amyloid beta peptide-induced neurotoxicity via extracellular signal-regulated kinase 1/2-dependent nuclear factor erythroid 2-related factor 2 activation. *Mol Pharmacol* 73, no. 6: 1785–95.

Wu, F., W. S. Poon, G. Lu, et al. 2009. Alpha-Synuclein knockdown attenuates MPP(+) induced mitochondrial dysfunction of SH-SY5Y cells. *Brain Res* 1292: 173–79.

Xi, Y. D., H. L. Yu, J. Ding, et al. 2012. Flavonoids protect cerebrovascular endothelial cells through Nrf2 and PI3K from beta-amyloid peptide-induced oxidative damage. *Curr Neurovasc Res* 9, no. 1: 32–41.

Xifro, X., J. M. Garcia-Martinez, D. Del Toro, et al. 2008. Calcineurin is involved in the early activation of NMDA-mediated cell death in mutant huntingtin knock-in striatal cells. *J Neurochem* 105, no. 5: 1596–612.

Xu, J., N. Zhong, H. Wang, et al. 2005. The Parkinson's disease-associated DJ-1 protein is a transcriptional co-activator that protects against neuronal apoptosis. *Hum Mol Genet* 14, no. 9: 1231–41.

Yanai, A., K. Huang, R. Kang, et al. 2006. Palmitoylation of huntingtin by HIP14 is essential for its trafficking and function. *Nat Neurosci* 9, no. 6: 824–31.

Yang, L., N. Y. Calingasan, E. J. Wille, et al. 2009. Combination therapy with coenzyme Q10 and creatine produces additive neuroprotective effects in models of Parkinson's and Huntington's diseases. *J Neurochem* 109, no. 5: 1427–39.

Young, F. B., S. L. Butland, S. S. Sanders, et al. 2012. Putting proteins in their place: palmitoylation in Huntington disease and other neuropsychiatric diseases. *Prog Neurobiol* 97, no. 2: 220–38.

Yuen, E. Y., J. Wei, P. Zhong, and Z. Yan. 2012. Disrupted GABAAR trafficking and synaptic inhibition in a mouse model of Huntington's disease. *Neurobiol Dis* 46, no. 2: 497–502.

Zambrano, S., A. J. Blanca, M. V. Ruiz-Armenta, et al. 2013. The renoprotective effect of L-carnitine in hypertensive rats is mediated by modulation of oxidative stress-related gene expression. *Eur J Nutr* 52, no. 6: 1649–59.

Zhang, H. N., J. F. Guo, D. He, et al. 2012. Lower serum UA levels in Parkinson's disease patients in the Chinese population. *Neurosci Lett* 514, no. 2: 152–55.

Zhang, S. M., M. A. Hernan, H. Chen, et al. 2002. Intakes of vitamins E and C, carotenoids, vitamin supplements, and PD risk. *Neurology* 59, no. 8: 1161–69.

Zhou, W., J. Schaack, W. M. Zawada, and C. R. Freed. 2002. Overexpression of human alpha-synuclein causes dopamine neuron death in primary human mesencephalic culture. *Brain Res* 926, nos. 1–2: 42–50.

Zhu, J., W. Yong, X. Wu, et al. 2008. Anti-inflammatory effect of resveratrol on TNF-alpha-induced MCP-1 expression in adipocytes. *Biochem Biophys Res Commun* 369, no. 2: 471–77.

Zou, Y., B. Hong, L. Fan, et al. 2013. Protective effect of puerarin against beta-amyloid-induced oxidative stress in neuronal cultures from rat hippocampus: involvement of the GSK-3beta/Nrf2 signaling pathway. *Free Radic Res* 47, no. 1: 55–63.

Zuccato, C., and E. Cattaneo. 2007. Role of brain-derived neurotrophic factor in Huntington's disease. *Prog Neurobiol* 81, nos. 5–6: 294–330.

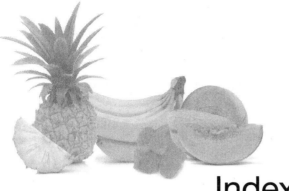

Index

Page numbers followed by *t* indicate tables.

About the Author

Kedar N. Prasad, Ph.D., former president of the International Society for Nutrition and Cancer, obtained a master's degree in zoology from the University of Bihar, Ranchi, India, and his Ph.D. degree in radiation biology from the University of Iowa, Iowa City, in 1963. He then attended the Brookhaven National Laboratory on Long Island for postdoctoral training before joining the Department of Radiology at the University of Colorado Health Sciences Center, where he became a professor in 1980. Later he was appointed director of the Center for Vitamins and Cancer Research at the University of Colorado School of Medicine. In 1982 he was invited by the Nobel Prize Committee to nominate a candidate for the Nobel Prize in medicine, and in 1999 he was selected to deliver the Harold Harper Lecture at the meeting of the American College of Advancement in Medicine.

His published papers and articles have appeared in illustrious publications such as *Science, Nature,* and *Proceedings of the National Academy of Sciences of the United States of America* (PNAS). He is also the author of several book chapters and twenty-five books, including *Fighting Cancer with Vitamins and Antioxidants.* A member of several professional organizations, he serves as an ad-hoc member of various study sections of the National Institutes of Health (NIH) and has consistently obtained NIH grants for his research.

Kedar N. Prasad is frequently an invited speaker at national and international meetings on nutrition and cancer. He began researching the effects of radiation on animal models in 1963. Over the next thirty-five years he continued his biological research at three major universities and national research labs, studying the relationships between micronutrients, cancer, and radiation and focusing on the effects that micronutrients have on human cells and the manner in which they interact with mainstream medical therapies for many common diseases. He found that certain combinations of micronutrients when taken in conjunction with standard treatments, such as chemotherapy, enhanced and complemented the effects of these traditional therapies. The findings inspired him to further his research to determine the effects that these micronutrient combinations might have on other diseases and on human health in general.

His present research interests are in the areas of radiation protection, nutrition and cancer, and nutrition and neurological diseases, particularly Alzheimer's disease and Parkinson's disease. He is the former chief scientific officer of the Premier Micronutrient Corporation, which produces antioxidant micronutrient formulations to promote a healthy lifestyle, and he is an independent consultant to nutrition industries.

BOOKS OF RELATED INTEREST

Fight Alzheimer's with Vitamins and Antioxidants
by Kedar N. Prasad, Ph.D.

Treat Concussion, TBI, and PTSD with Vitamins and Antioxidants
by Kedar N. Prasad, Ph.D.

Fight Heart Disease with Vitamins and Antioxidants
by Kedar N. Prasad, Ph.D.

Fighting Cancer with Vitamins and Antioxidants
by Kedar N. Prasad, Ph.D. and K. Che Prasad, M.S., M.D.

Adaptogens in Medical Herbalism
Elite Herbs and Natural Compounds for Mastering Stress,
Aging, and Chronic Disease
by Donald R. Yance Jr., CN, MH, RH(AHG)

The High Blood Pressure Solution
A Scientifically Proven Program for Preventing Strokes and Heart Disease
by Richard Moore, M.D., Ph.D.

Herbs for Healthy Aging
Natural Prescriptions for Vibrant Health
by David Hoffmann, FNIMH, AHG

The Neurofeedback Solution
How to Treat Autism, ADHD, Anxiety,
Brain Injury, Stroke, PTSD, and More
by Stephen Larsen, Ph.D.

INNER TRADITIONS • BEAR & COMPANY
P.O. Box 388
Rochester, VT 05767
1-800-246-8648
www.InnerTraditions.com

Or contact your local bookseller